Cases & Applications for An Introduction to Human Services

Seventh Edition

CASES & APPLICATIONS FOR AN INTRODUCTION TO HUMAN SERVICES

SEVENTH EDITION

Tricia McClam
University of Tennessee

Marianne Woodside
University of Tennessee

The authors contributed equally to the writing of this book.

BROOKS/COLE
CENGAGE Learning™

Australia • Brazil • Japan • Korea • Mexico • Singapore • Spain • United Kingdom • United States

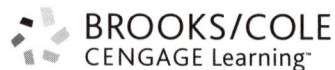

BROOKS/COLE
CENGAGE Learning™

Cases & Applications for An Introduction to Human Services, Seventh Edition
Tricia McClam and Marianne Woodside

Acquisitions Editor: Seth Dobrin

Developmental Editor: Arwen Petty

Editorial Assistant: Suzanna Kincaid

Media Editor: Dennis Fitzgerald

Marketing Assistant: Gurpeet Saran

Marketing Communications Manager: Tami Strang

Content Project Management: PreMediaGlobal

Design Director: Rob Hugel

Senior Art Director: Caryl Gorska

Senior Print Buyer: Linda Hsu

Senior Rights Specialist: Dean Dauphinais

Production Service: PreMediaGlobal

Photo Research: PreMediaGlobal

Text Research: PreMediaGlobal

Copy Editor: Patrice Titterington

Cover Designer: Lisa Buckley

Cover Image: Diana Ong/Superstock/Getty Images

Compositor: PreMediaGlobal

For product information and technology assistance, contact us at **Cengage Learning Customer & Sales Support, 1-800-354-9706**.

For permission to use material from this text or product, submit all requests online at **www.cengage.com/permissions**. Further permissions questions can be e-mailed to **permissionrequest@cengage.com**.

Library of Congress Control Number: 2010939069

Student Edition:

ISBN-13: 978-0-8400-3447-2

ISBN-10: 0-8400-3447-4

Brooks/Cole
20 Davis Drive
Belmont, CA 94002-3098
USA

Cengage Learning is a leading provider of customized learning solutions with office locations around the globe, including Singapore, the United Kingdom, Australia, Mexico, Brazil, and Japan. Locate your local office at **www.cengage.com/global**.

Cengage Learning products are represented in Canada by **Nelson Education, Ltd.**

To learn more about Brooks/Cole, visit **www.cengage.com/brookscole**
Purchase any of our products at your local college store or at our preferred online store **www.cengagebrain.com**.

CONTENTS

PREFACE

This text was written for you, the student. In our combined 50-plus years of teaching human services, our students have told us time and again that they value opportunities to apply what they have learned from their textbooks, class discussions, and lectures. For this reason, we have written *Cases & Applications for An Introduction to Human Services* to supplement *Introduction to Human Services, 7th ed.* Its purpose is to provide you with opportunities, activities, and exercises to reinforce the important concepts introduced in the textbook. Each chapter in this supplement corresponds to a chapter in *Introduction to Human Services*. For example, Chapter 1 in this supplement reflects the content of Chapter 1 in the textbook. These matched chapters have the same number and name.

You can follow several steps to maximize your learning as you use this supplement. We recommend that you first carefully read the chapter in *Introduction to Human Services* before you turn to the corresponding chapter in the supplement. The textbook chapters introduce and explore introductory human service concepts; the supplement chapters build upon this information as they focus on application, reflection, and further study. The components of each chapter follow:

- The first exercise introduces you to the content and focus of the chapter.
- The second exercise asks you to reflect on your own experiences as they relate to the chapter topic.
- Key concepts from the textbook chapter are then briefly reviewed. At this point, if any concepts are unfamiliar to you, you may want to return to the textbook chapter for a more complete discussion of the concept.
- Following the review of concepts is a section that provides a context for the client or case study that is next. For example, in Chapter 7 you will read about Puerto Rican culture before meeting Gloria, a Puerto Rican woman trying to balance family needs with her education needs in order to support her family.

- Next are questions to facilitate your application of key concepts to the client or case study.
- You will then read another perspective of the study. This section may be the perspective of an agency board member, an agency supervisor, or an ethicist. Coupled with additional questions, this "real world" perspective provides an opportunity for further reflection and discussion.
- Finally, we hope that each chapter will stimulate you to explore further human service client groups, dilemmas, problems, and professionals. To assist you in this effort, each chapter concludes with related books, movies, and Web sites.

The cases presented in this supplement may evoke some strong reactions from you and your classmates. Because the clients are realistically portrayed, you may question their language, values, and behavior; you may feel uncomfortable reading about some of these clients. Confronting your own strong reactions, opinions, and biases is part of the learning process, especially as you discover different types of clients and client groups. These cases allow you to demonstrate respect for clients, regardless of their religious affiliation, language, ethnicity, beliefs, or behaviors. Discussion of the cases with classmates provides you with the opportunity to demonstrate acceptance and tolerance for classmates whose opinions differ from yours.

Features new to this text are updated references and ideas for further study, including books, movies, and Web sites. We have also updated material to coincide with the changes that appear in the seventh edition of *Introduction to Human Services*, so that this text will continue as a supplement to the concepts introduced in that text. And of course, you will find many other resources for further study as you increase your knowledge about these topics. We hope you will share them with us.

We designed this supplement for use by individuals and groups, in and out of class. Instructors will vary in their use of the supplement. However it is used, we hope it stimulates your thinking about human services; promotes reflection about your own experiences, knowledge, and skills; and provides opportunities to practice what you are learning in your human service courses. As you work your way through the supplement, other questions, exercises, and activities may occur to you. Again, please share them with us!

As always, undertakings such as the writing of this text involve many good people. We wish to extend our thanks to our friends at Brooks/Cole, especially Seth Dobrin, Editor, and Suzanna Kincaid, Editorial Assistant.

We always find feedback from reviewers productive and we are indebted to the following individuals who were so helpful in refining the contents: Professor Jody Weigel, Kirkland Community College; Professor Susan E. Claxton, Georgia Highlands College; and Professor David Callhoun, Columbia College.

And finally, we thank our families and our colleagues for their interest in and support of our work.

Cases & Applications for An Introduction to Human Services

Seventh Edition

AN INTRODUCTION TO HUMAN SERVICES

Defining *human services* is a challenge because it is a complex term. Some people think of human services as the name of an agency, an organization, or an academic major in college. Others consider it a profession or a position. Yet another way to define human services is what a human service professional actually does to help others. The purpose of this first chapter is to assist your exploration of the term *human services* and the important concepts that will help you understand it.

The chapter begins with an exercise that connects the content of Chapter 1 in *Introduction to Human Services, 7th ed.* with this chapter. The second exercise introduces you to the focus of this chapter, the elderly. A list of key ideas and their definitions follows. A case study about Beth and Ruth, her elderly stepmother, illustrates how the terms introduced in this chapter apply to the "real" world. Understanding each term and its application to the case of Beth and Ruth will increase your knowledge of human services. The case study is followed by questions to consider as you develop an understanding of human services. Finally, a discussion of how the case relates to the larger world of human services from a human service professional's perspective concludes the chapter. Additional resources are listed for further exploration.

INTRODUCTION

The purpose of this exercise is to assist you in thinking about human service problems, participants, organizations, and issues. Select a news story about the elderly that reflects a human service problem, and follow this story in the newspaper, on television, and in other media for two days.

1.   Describe the situation you are following in the media.

_____

_____

_____

_____

_____

2.   What is the problem?

_____

_____

_____

_____

3.   Who are the participants? What different perspectives do the participants have?

_____

_____

_____

_____

_____

4.   How is the situation resolved?

_____

_____

_____

_____

_____

5.   How well or how poorly do you think the media portrayed the situation? Why?

_____

_____

_____

_____

_____

EXERCISE: WHAT ABOUT YOU?

Think about an elderly person in your life—a grandparent, a neighbor; a church, mosque, or temple member; or an acquaintance. How would you describe his or her life, needs, problems, or challenges? You might want to think about issues such as housing, transportation, medical care, or family. Based on what you know about human services, describe services that would be helpful to the person you have selected.

_____

_____

_____

_____

_____

KEY IDEAS

Central to understanding human services is knowing and understanding its purpose. Why does society have human services? What do these services accomplish? How are they delivered? To answer these questions, five important ideas that underlie the human service profession are explored.

PROBLEMS IN LIVING

This phrase describes a set of circumstances that present difficulties for a person. Examples include needs for food, clothing, health care, housing, employment, safety, and positive interpersonal relationships. In human services, problems in living are addressed by focusing on the client, the environment (including other people), and the interaction between the two in order to promote the individual's self-sufficiency.

INTERDISCIPLINARY NATURE

This term refers to the contributions of different fields of study to the development and understanding of human services. Disciplines that complement human services are anthropology (the study of the role of culture and its relationship to human behavior and the environment), psychology (the study of how people think, feel, and behave), and sociology (the study of the elements of life that affect living such as family structure, gender, ethnicity, and poverty). The blend of these three disciplines supports the work of human service professionals.

COLLABORATION

Working with other professionals to access needed services for clients is one way human service professionals cope with limited resources, cutbacks in services, shifting political beliefs and bureaucracy, and the emergence of new client groups. In addition to working with other professionals, human service providers also establish partnerships with their clients. Actively engaging the client in problem identification, goal setting, and plan development promotes the client's self-sufficiency and the development of problem-solving skills.

NETWORKING

Learning about other agencies and establishing relationships with other professionals are ways service providers work together to meet client needs. These connections assist in identifying needed services, making referrals, and following up service delivery.

CASE MANAGEMENT

This term refers to one method of human service delivery that has a dual focus: providing services and coordinating the services provided by other professionals and agencies. Coordination means arranging for services from other agencies, advocating for clients, allocating resources, and providing quality assurance. Collaboration and networking skills enhance the helper's ability to coordinate services.

GENERALIST APPROACH

This concept describes an approach to service delivery that is fundamental to human services. Human service professionals assume a variety of responsibilities in various settings with diverse client groups. This approach requires preparation in the core knowledge, values, and skills common across client groups, settings, and job functions. Examples of this concept include interviewing, referring, and developing plans.

EXERCISE: YOU AND HUMAN SERVICES

This exercise will help you refine your definition of human services. Before you answer these questions, review your response to the exercise "What About You?" at the beginning of the chapter.

1. Which needs, problems, or challenges illustrate the problems in living concept?

_____

_____

_____

_____

_____

_____

_____

2. What are the advantages of collaboration in human services to this elderly person's situation?

_____

_____

_____

_____

_____

_____

_____

3. Provide examples of how each of the following might be implemented to provide services to your friend or relative:

Networking

_____

_____

_____

_____

_____

_____

_____

Case management

_____

_____

_____

_____

_____

_____

_____

FOCUS: CARING FOR THE ELDERLY

One of the best ways to develop your understanding of human services is to learn about the serious social and economic challenges that people face, especially here in the United States. In this section, you will read about the problems Americans encounter in supporting the rapidly expanding population of the elderly. The seriousness of the problem is documented and the question "Who will care for the elderly?" is explored. You will then meet Beth and her husband Tim and think about some difficulties they face with them. Beth's father has just died, leaving Ruth, his widow and Beth's stepmother, to continue life alone.

Demographic projections reflect the continued increase in the U.S. population of those in late adulthood. Although the statistics of the 2010 U.S. Census have not been made available at this writing, projections are that this population will be more diverse, female, and is projected to live much longer than ever before (U.S. Census Bureau, 2009). Many individuals reaching these older ages are living in poverty and do not have any "safety net" of family and friends. Women are more likely to be widowed and living alone. The centenarians (individuals over 100 years of age) are the fastest growing segment of the population.

As individuals age, they experience the age discrimination that illustrates this culture's lack of respect for the elderly. There are also some declines in vision, hearing, and performance of physical and mental reaction time. Attention span diminishes. Intelligence and mental abilities also change. Older individuals cannot perform tasks as quickly and their ability to analyze figures often decreases. In balance, there develops a wisdom that combines intuition, experience, and knowledge of life experiences. Aging can also signal a decline of social interaction and interest in the larger world. Many older individuals face the death of a spouse or death of their own children. Their social world changes as their friends become debilitated or die. Eventually individuals must consider their own mortality (Weiten, Lloyd, Dunn, & Hammer, 2009).

According to projections, the experience of aging will change as the baby boomers enter late adulthood. Some will focus on vocational retraining rather than retiring. Baby boomers will be on the move rather than staying at home. They will practice excellent nutrition, exercise, and maintain good health care. Aging will also change as technological and research advancements continue to provide new procedures, protocols, and treatments to extend longevity and quality of life. There remains, however, an aging population that is poor, without social support, and suffering ill health. Many may delay the aging process, but eventually they too will need the support and care from others.

From the human service perspective, concern for the elderly generates four questions: 1) What services are needed? 2) How much will the services cost? 3) Who will pay for the services? 4) Who will provide these services? With the growth in the number of individuals projected to live longer lives, demand for services in this age group will increase. Their needs will reflect the demand for the following services: financial assistance; health and mental health services; social and community support; rehabilitation, mobility, and independent living; housing alternatives and environmental modifications; education and employment assistance; and leisure and recreational opportunities.

As the number of the oldest old increases, much of the responsibility for care falls to their own adult children. These adult children are in their middle years, often still involved in raising families of their own. Because this middle generation is trying to meet both the needs of their own children and their parents, they are often referred to as the "sandwich generation." About 25 percent of Americans are in this sandwich generation (Abaya, n.d.). This term refers to the pressures members of this group feel as their responsibilities for providing care to others increases.

Within a family three generations need support: children, parents, and grandparents. Each generation has its own set of needs. Because of limited resources, many needs go unmet. For example, children, parents, and elderly parents all require social support. Children want the security of their family and want their parents to be available for them; in other words, they want their parents' time and attention. Teenagers want the flexibility and time to be with their friends. Those in middle adulthood often need a time for solitude, with few demands from others. Elderly parents wish to retain their connections to their previous lives and need emotional support and interaction with those for whom they care. Parents, sandwiched between children and their own parents, have difficulty making time to care for both. And they often sacrifice getting what they need while trying to meet the needs of others.

With additional pressures of work and care for the home, many times those in the sandwich generation only have the time and energy to respond to crises. Therefore, children do not receive the support they need because parents are also caring for elderly parents. Teens are left unsupervised. Elderly parents miss the interaction and outside stimulation with others that could enhance their quality of life. These families are experiencing an increased set of problems and need support from the human service delivery system.

CASE STUDY: MEET BETH AND RUTH

List of Characters

Beth—a young woman returning home for her father's funeral. She is married to Tim, a house painter, and is the mother of two children.

Tim—Beth's husband

Ruth Helms—Beth's stepmother, a retired beautician

Dr. Cynthia Cable—an eye specialist

Harry Flannery—a caseworker who has experience with clients with vision problems

The Case

BETH *Driving down Main Street in their hometown, Tim and Beth look sadly at the rundown, empty buildings along the street where they once used to cruise and hang out. The old drugstore soda shop where they met after school stands empty, the windows are yellowed and cracked. They are both lost in memories of how this area used to be when they were young. They remember little shops and family-run businesses scattered up and down the street, the ice cream shop on the corner, the* Five and Dime, *and the old department store before it burned in the fire of 1967.*

The old brick buildings, now rundown, are still standing, but they are empty. It isn't really a surprise, Beth thought to herself. The decay of this area has been slow. The bustling little town of 2,500 survived two fires that burned much of the

commercial town to the ground, but they have taken their toll. The small family-owned businesses could not afford to start over. Then, when the coal mines became automated, their layoffs just about closed the town. Tim and Beth had worked hard to leave and pursue a better life elsewhere. It was not easy getting the education to go to college in a town where over half of the high school population did not graduate and college prep classes were scarce.

Neither Beth nor Tim were able to go to college, but they did move away for a fresh start. Beth now works in a bakery factory and has a responsible position on the night shift. She began as an hourly worker many years ago, but is now salaried. In some respects, Tim has not been as fortunate as Beth. He has moved from job to job in the past ten years. He has been employed as a house painter for more than six months. Tim makes an hourly wage and always has work because of the growth in the city in which they live. As Tim and Beth continue to gaze at their hometown streets, they realize the only people who are left are the elderly who have lived here all their lives, people who work in the nearby factory, and others who are out of work and living on government subsidies.

It is the first time Tim and Beth have been home in eight years. They always meant to come home before now but somehow they just never found the time. They always had some excuse, like work or childcare responsibilities, but they both knew the truth. Beth had a falling out with her father years ago. It was a result of her father's marriage to a woman Beth did not particularly like. Beth's mother had died when she was very young and this woman was considered an unwelcome addition to her family.

The woman, Ruth Helms, was a beautician, and had cut Beth's hair when she was growing up from time to time. Miss Helms had been unfeeling and hateful, often embarrassing Beth in front of others in the shop. She was nothing like Beth's sweet and giving mother. How could her father love this woman? Beth had wondered. When her father announced his plans to marry Ruth, the embarrassment of his marriage was more than Beth could handle. How could he do this to her mother? How could he do this to her? And why did he have to marry this woman? Beth simply could not bring herself to forgive her father.

Issues Beth Faces on Her Return Home

- Deterioration of her hometown
- Death of her father
- Unresolved anger toward her father
- Face-to-face interaction with her stepmother, Ruth

Although those bridges were supposedly mended years ago, Beth still could not stand the thought of this woman in her family's home, in her mother's place. She had stayed in touch with her father and Ruth, and they had been to visit her, but Beth always felt they made judgments about her life in the city. Because Tim's parents had moved away shortly after he graduated from high school, it was easy for him to find excuses not to go back, too.

None of that mattered now as, like it or not, Tim and Beth were here. They had no choice. Years of hard labor in the coal mines had finally claimed Beth's father. Although he had been retired for years, he had finally lost the struggle against black lung disease. Now they were back in town, not to visit or to make peace, but to attend her father's funeral.

The car pulled up slowly to Beth's childhood home. At least it looked much the same. Her dad had always maintained the house, taking great pride in the appearance of his home. The yard had recently been mowed by the boy down the street. The paint still looked fresh, although the house had not been painted recently. It was a small but cozy dwelling. Tears welled up in Beth's eyes as memories of her father and her childhood occupied her thoughts. The house looked so much the same that she almost expected to see her father appear at the front door to greet them. This was the only place, it seemed, that time had not decayed in the town.

Instead, Beth's stepmother, Ruth, greeted them at the door. Beth was shocked when she saw her. Somehow, Ruth didn't seem to be the same wicked witch that Beth had always known. She appeared old and broken, not the fiery old bat Beth had remembered. Ruth was now old and alone. In spite of herself, Beth felt sorry for this pitiful old woman. They all sat at the kitchen table and tried to make small talk while they waited to leave for the funeral. Beth began to feel a strange sort of closeness to Ruth, the closeness of a shared loss.

The funeral and graveside service went smoothly. Ruth sat stoically while barely even blinking. She stared straight ahead. Beth felt sick to her stomach. She did not know if she would be able to make it through the entire service. All of these years she had been so angry with her father. Only now did she realize how much she had missed him. She wanted to blame all the missed time on Ruth, but somehow blame and bitterness seemed so petty right now. Ruth was obviously hurting as much as she was. Ruth had truly loved her father, just as Beth had. That was something Beth was trying to hold on to now. Beth looked up at Tim and he quickly placed his arm around her. She did not have to say anything to her husband. He almost always automatically knew what she was feeling, just from a look. It had been that way ever since high school when they first started dating. Thank God he was here now with her. She didn't think she could handle this on her own. At least Daddy won't have to be sick anymore, she thought, as she placed a rose on his coffin.

After the funeral, the family returned home. Tim and Beth had planned to leave early the next morning. Tim needed to get back to work, and the children were staying with the neighbors. They were emotionally and physically exhausted after the day's events. The long drive and the intense emotions of the funeral had worn them out. They all sat around the table filled with food that neighbors and friends had brought, but no one ate. They sat in an uncomfortable silence, not knowing what to say or where to start. Suddenly Ruth burst into tears. She was deeply grieving for her husband, but more than that she was frightened. Through her deep sobs she began telling Beth and Tim her fears.

She was slowly going blind and already her vision was severely impaired. She had had to quit her work at the beauty shop. The diagnosis was retinitis pigmentosa. In another year or two she would be completely blind. Only Ray had known because she had not wanted pity from relatives or friends. Now Ruth did not know how she would manage without him. She had always thought that he would be there to take care of her once her sight was completely gone. Even if he had black lung disease, he could be her eyes. She described a lot of other worries and fears about life without Ray, including how to pay for the funeral. Beth had been so caught up in her own grieving that she had not realized what her father's death meant to Ruth.

After talking with Tim, Beth decided that she should stay a little longer and help Ruth decide where to go from here. No matter what her personal feelings for this woman were, her father had loved her and now it was Beth's responsibility to see that she was taken care of. Her father would have wanted that. All of Ruth's family had long been dead. She had some friends, but most of them were also in their later years and had physical and financial problems of their own. They would all do what they could but, in most cases, that was minimal. Ray was all that Ruth had. Now Beth was all that she had. What an ironic twist of fate for all involved.

The next morning Tim left for home, and Beth called her boss to ask for a week's vacation. Her boss only moderately understood but finally relented. Beth then began skimming the local weekly paper looking for advertisements or information about any services that might be of help to Ruth. They needed someone to help them with the dire financial situation. Beth and Tim had $600 in the bank and $200 in savings, not nearly enough to pay for the funeral or other expenses, and Ruth had little savings of her own. They finally found the telephone number of Ray's employer, and made an appointment to talk to Mr. Blank, the personnel and benefits director. Both Beth and Ruth would visit him the next day.

Ruth's Circumstances

• Diagnosis of retinitis pigmentosa	• Lack of transportation
• Financial insecurity	• Few support services
• Loss of her spouse, Ray	• Little medical support in town
• Dependence on Beth	

Beth next looked for services that might help Ruth with her physical problems, but she found nothing. The paper consisted mostly of church and local high school news. Beth asked Ruth if she had been seeing old Dr. Barton about her vision problem. Ruth told her that Dr. Barton had died three years ago and that his son had taken over his practice. Now, young Dr. Barton was planning to leave and go to a larger city to start a practice because he could not make ends meet in this small town. In fact, Ray had been taking Ruth into a nearby town to see a vision specialist the last few months before his death. Ruth lost her driver's license when she could no longer pass the eye test, so she could not drive and had no way of getting into town on her own. Not only that, it was also becoming more difficult for her to find her way around unfamiliar places without getting lost or running into something. Beth began to realize that she had very little understanding of the extent of Ruth's disease and needed to learn more about it if she was going to help Ruth. She was afraid the only alternative might be a nursing home, but she did not know how they would afford it. All of her friends either had or expected to have their parents living in their homes. Unfortunately, for many of them it was not a welcome situation.

According to Ruth, after Dr. Barton's departure, there would be no medical doctor or clinic in their town. Ruth was concerned about herself and all her friends who needed medical care. They were all getting along in years, and the nearest doctor would be an hour away. There would be no one to write prescriptions or provide emergency care. Ruth tried to make light of the situation and told Beth that it was not so bad because she had felt funny seeing a doctor who was so young, but Beth could tell how upset she really was about her situation.

Beth decided that day to telephone Dr. Cynthia Cable, the specialist who had diagnosed Ruth's eye disease. Beth asked Dr. Cable to explain the disease and what Beth could do for Ruth. Beth learned the following facts:

- Retinitis pigmentosa is a hereditary, degenerative disease that slowly robs its victims of their eyesight.
- It strikes all ages of people, usually starting in youth, but it is not typically diagnosed until the later years because the darkening and blurring of the eyesight is such a slow process.
- Most patients, after being diagnosed, can recall events that happened to them throughout their lives that are signs of the disease, but these signs are usually attributed to nearsightedness, clumsiness, or sometimes just mere stupidity.

Beth really did not understand much of this medical information. She had little exposure to medical advice or discussions. Her own clinic served so many people that there was no time for conversation with medical personnel. Ruth was in the later stages of this disease, the doctor explained. Unfortunately, retinitis pigmentosa was incurable, and there was not much more medically that the doctor could do for Ruth. But a caseworker who specialized in degenerative blindness could help her learn to cope and meet her basic needs. She gave Beth the telephone number of a caseworker she knew. Beth was not sure what to do. How could she trust a stranger? She needed someone to provide services, not to talk about unrelated issues. Beth reluctantly called and arranged for an appointment for herself and Ruth for the next morning; she felt she had no alternative. She had to get back home to work and the children, and helping Ruth took her mind off her father for a little while and made her feel somewhat stronger.

RUTH   *Ruth reluctantly agreed to go to the appointment to see the caseworker. She was beginning to feel the loss of her independence already, and while she appreciated Beth's help, she felt very uncomfortable accepting help from a person who she knew had resented her all her life. Accepting help from anyone but Ray was new to Ruth. She was frightened that Beth might lock her up in a nursing home and forget about her. Ruth would have no grounds to contest that action if she could not take care of herself. She tried to push these thoughts out of her mind and believe that Beth was really trying to be of help, but the fact that Beth kept making decisions without even asking her kept this idea alive. There was a time, not too long ago, that Ruth would have exploded with anger at someone else making decisions for her, but now, she just did not have the energy to fight.*

The next morning Beth and Ruth arrived at the office of Harry Flannery, the caseworker. He was a bit overweight and gruff looking and Ruth did not much care for his looks or his manners. He pointed to two chairs for the women. He began by saying that he had read the medical report from Dr. Cable and had experience with this disease. The caseworker said that the prognosis was not good, that Ruth would probably be completely blind within a year and with the inevitable problems of aging, would be unable to live on her own. He felt that she had three options:

- She could hire a live-in companion.
- She could find a good retirement community.
- She could move in with a close relative or friend.

At this point, the caseworker paused. Ruth sat frozen, stunned by the amount of information and the way he rattled it off like some kind of checklist. She looked at Beth; they both felt uneasy with this situation. He went on to say that when they had made their choice he could refer them to some retirement centers or live-in care agencies. Once again he paused, but both women still sat silent and bewildered. He dismissed them by saying that he could see they both needed time to think about their choices. The caseworker asked them to let him know their decision, and he would help them make the next move from there. The two women said "good-bye" and stood up to leave.

Ruth did not say a word all the way home. She was overwhelmed with the information they had received, and she thought Beth was, too. This appointment was not at all what they had hoped for. They came into the house and sat at the dining room table. Ruth began to cry. She knew Beth was both concerned about her and anxious to get home. Beth did not know what to do. She asked Ruth what she thought would be best for her. Ruth sobbed even harder. She said that she didn't have the money for a live-in companion. Ray was so sick before he died that he had not renewed their insurance policy, although he had meant to do this. Ruth had never worried about the finances before as Ray had always taken care of them. She also could not afford a retirement community, and the idea of a nursing home terrified her. She doubted she could afford the latter suggestion either.

Ruth's Options

- Nursing home
- Live-in companion
- Adult day care
- Living with relative or friend

BETH AND RUTH *Beth left the dining room and made tea for them both. When she returned, she asked Ruth about nursing homes. According to Ruth, there was only one nursing home in the town, and since half the town population was sickly and elderly, it had a long waiting list. Ruth had some friends who lived in the nursing home, or "retirement center," as they chose to call it. Her friends entered the nursing home because they were lonely and wanted companionship or they had minor problems that made them unable to be self-sufficient, but once there, something happened to them. All of a sudden these friends got old, really old, and most of the time they got sicker. Ruth believed that having someone do everything for you and treat you like you are old can quickly age someone. Ruth had always said that she would never let that happen to her. And some of her friends could not afford the home, so they moved in with their children. That situation did not always work well either. What choice did Ruth have now? Thoughts of living with Beth, who was both her closest family member now and the woman who two days ago could not stand her, was not an appealing thought.*

Beth's thoughts at this time were frantic. Reflecting upon Harry Flannery's suggestions, she considered hiring a live-in companion, locating adult day care services, finding a retirement community for Ruth, or moving Ruth in with a close relative or friend. Since there was so little money available, I suppose that means she will have to move in with us, Beth mused. She remembered that there was a nursing home here in this town. Shouldn't she and Ruth consider it as a possibility? Maybe they have special financial options for those who worked in the mines or for those who were related to the mine workers?

Deciding what to do about Ruth was more complicated than she thought it would be. Beth thought that she shouldn't leave until this situation is resolved because Ruth couldn't handle this on her own. Unfortunately, she felt that she could not stay much longer and lose her wages. Exhausted by the funeral, dealing with Ruth and her problems, and visiting the doctor and the caseworker, Beth decided to say nothing to Ruth now, preferring to call her husband Tim after dinner to discuss the options.

Case Questions

1. Identify the problems in living faced by Ruth and Beth. How does each experience these problems?

---

2. What is self-sufficiency for Ruth?

_____

_____

_____

_____

3. Describe Beth's thoughts and feelings about Ruth.

_____

_____

_____

_____

_____

_____

_____

4. Describe Ruth's thoughts and feelings about her own situation and her thoughts and feelings about Beth and the help she is providing.

_____

_____

_____

_____

_____

_____

_____

5. List the human service professionals involved in this case and define their professional expertise.

_____

_____

_____

_____

_____

_____

_____

6. Describe any evidence that collaboration occurs.

_____

_____

_____

_____

_____

_____

_____

7. What do these human service professionals do that is helpful? Not helpful?

_____

_____

_____

_____

_____

_____

_____

8. Is Beth part of the sandwich generation? Explain.

_____

_____

_____

_____

_____

_____

_____

The following four questions focus on services:

9. What services does Ruth need?

_____

_____

_____

_____

_____

_____

_____

_____

10. How would you find information about these services?

_____

_____

_____

_____

_____

_____

_____

11. Is there informal help that could be accessed?

_____

_____

_____

_____

_____

_____

_____

12. Can you think of other questions that need to be addressed in order to provide services to Ruth?

_____

_____

_____

_____

_____

_____

_____

EXERCISE: YOU AS THE HUMAN SERVICE PROFESSIONAL

Now that you have increased your awareness of some basic human service concepts and are familiar with Ruth and Beth's dilemma, answer the following
questions:

1. What is your reaction to this case?

_____

_____

_____

_____

_____

_____

_____

2. What do you think are the challenges working with clients in late adulthood?

_____

_____

_____

_____

_____

_____

_____

3. Suppose Beth and Ruth come to see you rather than the caseworker Harry
    Flannery. Describe how you would conduct the meeting.

_____

_____

_____

_____

_____

_____

_____

_____

4. In your opinion, what is the best way to resolve the problems facing Beth and
    Ruth?

_____

_____

_____

_____

_____

_____

_____

5. What qualities or characteristics do you have that would help you work effec-
    tively with Beth and Ruth?

_____

_____

_____

_____

_____

_____

_____

6. What difficulties would you encounter?

_____

_____

_____

_____

_____

_____

_____

ANOTHER PERSPECTIVE: BROOK DICKERSON

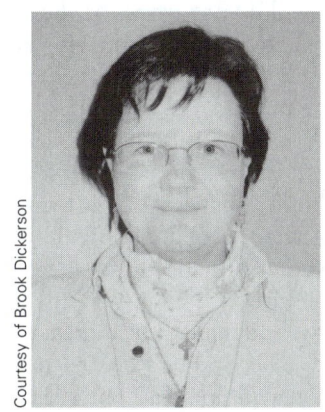

Courtesy of Brook Dickerson

Brook H. Dickerson's position as manager of the senior nutrition program at the local Council on Aging makes her uniquely qualified to provide a practitioner's perspective on Beth and Ruth's situation. In this position, Brook is responsible for serving meals to approximately 1,000 seniors each weekday.

Brook's academic background includes a bachelor's degree. in business and a master's degree in human relations. Her work background is varied and includes positions with the U.S. Departments of Defense and State and as a senior vice president at a bank. She has also worked in retail merchandising and management.

In this case study Beth and her stepmother Ruth are up against some real issues. Not only must they deal with the mental and emotional trauma of Beth's father's death, but the lack of a real relationship between the two of them is another stumbling block. Add to these issues, Ruth's loss of independence due to her physical health and aging and Beth's family and career issues, and the two of them have far more on their plates than is healthy for either one.

So where to start? I suggest that we deal with some of the more obvious, practical issues first. Beth and Ruth have several options.

- Beth can call the Social Security office to see what kind of income her stepmother can expect from her husband's Social Security every month, and set up an appointment (if needed) to update the paperwork so Ruth can receive a monthly check.
- Next, Beth should call her father's prior employer to see if he had a retirement pension, and if those benefits will come to Ruth now that Beth's father is dead.
- Beth should call the local United Mine Workers Union to see if her dad had any insurance, union benefits, or black lung disability payments that Ruth might be entitled to receive.
- Explore food stamps for Ruth.
- Immediate assistance may be available from local food pantries, if there are any in this community.

An array of services are also available at the local Office on Aging. There is one in every county in the United States. Beth should see what types of services are available in Ruth's small town. It is likely that the local Office on Aging will only provide two or three services, but even those might be helpful to Ruth.

- Meals on Wheels—most of the time, cost is negligible to low-income participants; however, availability varies.
- Transportation to medical appointments and the area hospital. Amounts and service costs vary in each state and county.
- A senior center often provides opportunities for socializing and other activities.
- Congregate Meals—a low-cost, cafeteria-style lunch service is available at the senior center.

Unfortunately, there may be a drawback to visiting the senior center; how would Ruth get there? The center is probably not close enough for Ruth to walk and transportation may or may not be available to transport her there. So, as with the other services, Beth needs to get all the information she can. She needs to become informed quickly so that she and her stepmother can make some informed choices about what services are best for Ruth.

Now to some of the less concrete issues that Beth and her stepmother face. They both need counseling for grief, loss, and relationship building. The Office on Aging may have some resources in this area, or if Ruth is a member of a religious or civic group, they may be able to help. Many organizations have formal or informal support groups or pastoral care. (Note: Beth should look for a similar service, or regular counseling for herself and her husband, Tim, when she gets back home. Ruth's situation is not going to go away and will only increase in difficulty over time. Beth will need to deal with grief over her father's death, and the guilt, resentment, and frustration that Ruth's situation will create. Tim will need to learn to be supportive and accepting of the circumstances in which his wife finds herself, and together they will need to help their children work through the changes that Ruth's situation will bring to their family life.)

PLAN OF ACTION

The results Beth finds from her research of available services will play a large part in the short- and long-term decisions that must be made for her stepmother's care. Beth and Ruth should make these decisions together, as much as possible. This collaboration will enable Ruth to have some control over what is happening to her (she has lost independence already). Although given her current emotional state, the extent to which Ruth is able to help make these decisions is unclear. But Beth must try to consider Ruth's thoughts, feelings, and choices, because her stepmother has a right to choose what her future holds.

Should Beth opt to move her stepmother to the city where she lives? I do NOT recommend that at this point, there will be a lot more resources available in the city where she lives. The local Office on Aging should be Beth's first phone call and a primary resource for researching available services, and helping her take advantage of them on behalf of Ruth. Services might include senior housing, social worker assistance, homemaker service grocery shopping and errand service, meals (either Congregate Meals or Meals on Wheels), food pantry delivery, senior centers, transportation to doctor and hospital appointments, low income energy assistance, and help with Medicare, wills, conservatorship, and other legal issues.

SHORT-TERM RECOMMENDATION

My short-term recommendation is to keep Ruth in her current home in town. Persuade Ruth to tell her friends, members of her religious community or social group, and others about her physical condition; enlist their help. Local friends and resources can help with meals, daily check-ins, and occasional transport until Social Security, the Office on Aging, food stamps, and the other services that they have arranged can fill in those gaps.

Beth needs to get back to her job in the city ASAP or risk losing it. When she returns, she needs to find some counseling support for herself and/or her family. She will also need to investigate the services that are available for Ruth in her city, in case the two of them decide that moving to Beth's town is the best for both of them in the long term. I would NOT recommend that Beth move Ruth into her home. Both of them must resolve all of the old issues and develop a genuine respect and love for each other. Otherwise, Beth is likely to wreck her marriage, her family, and her career by moving Ruth into her home.

LONG-TERM RECOMMENDATION

If Beth chooses to move her stepmother to the city where she and her family live, they both need to take some time before they make the move. The longer time they both have to work through their grief, personal issues, and Ruth's eventual dependence on Beth, the better. Beth will need to plan ahead, put as many services as possible in place before moving her stepmother to the city, and make the move when she and Tim can take a little time off from their jobs.

If Beth chooses not to move Ruth to the city, or if Ruth adamantly refuses the move (she is still an independent person with the right to choose her own path), then hard choices will need to be made. Ruth's eyesight will fail, she will be blind and unable to care for herself, and at that time long-term care will be her only option. The house will need to be sold to pay for long-term care if they don't decide to sell it before that time, and after that Medicare will take up the payments for Ruth's placement in a care facility.

EXERCISE: THE LAST WORD

You have the opportunity to have the last word on the terms introduced and the case study presented. Based upon what you have learned in this chapter, answer the following questions.

1. When you think about what you have read about human services in this chapter, what stands out for you?

    _____

    _____

    _____

    _____

2. How did the chapter change your ideas and understanding about what human services is?

    _____

    _____

    _____

    _____

3. How will you use the information in this chapter in your own life and work?

_____

_____

_____

_____

4. What unanswered questions remain for you?

_____

_____

_____

_____

FOR FURTHER STUDY

BOOKS

Ellis, Neenah. (2002). *If I live to be 100: Lessons from the centenarians*. New York: Crown. Author interviews Americans at least 100 years old describing life in the final years.

Feldman, E., & Ludfke, I. (2009). *Living for the elderly: A design manual*. New York: Birkhauser Basic. Innovative types of housing, barrier-free building, and advanced systems of care are among the contributions of architects and builder to quality living for seniors.

Lieberman, Trudy (Ed.). (2000). *Consumer Reports complete guide to health services for seniors: What your family needs to know about finding and financing Medicare, assisted living, nursing homes, home care, adult day care*. New York: Three Rivers. The title of this guide lists the topics that are important to seniors and their families.

MOVIES

About Schmidt (2002). Director: Alexander Payne. Starring: Jack Nicholson, Kathy Bates, Dermot Mulroney, Hope Davis. Jack Nicholson plays a recently retired actuary who suddenly loses his wife. As he travels to his daughter's wedding, he finds most of his assumptions about life shaken.

On Golden Pond (1981). Director: Mark Rydell. Starring: Henry Fonda, Katharine Hepburn, Jane Fonda. Norman Thayer, a retired professor, and his wife, Ethel, are summering at their home on Golden Pond. Their daughter, Chelsea, comes to visit, bringing her fiancé and his son, Billy. Billy stays with Norman and Ethel while Chelsea and her fiancé travel to Europe. The plot focuses on Norman's struggle with aging, the development of a relationship between Norman and Billy, and the long-going tensions between Chelsea and Norman.

Something's Got to Give (2003). Director: Nancy Meyers. Starring: Jack Nicholson, Diane Keaton. A soon-to-be senior citizen falls in love with an accomplished women closer to his age.

WEB SITES

Explore the web to learn more about the following:

The Older Americans Act Nutrition Program

retinitis pigmentosa

Administration on Aging

AmericanAssociation of Retired Persons

National Institute on Aging

aging

housing problems

case management

social problems

elderly

sandwich generation

helping professions

unemployment

REFERENCES

Abaya, C. (n.d.). *The sandwich generation.* Retrieved from http://www.thesandwichgeneration.com/.

U.S. Census Bureau. (2009). *An aging world: 2008.* Retrieved from http://www.census.gov/Press-Release/www/releases/archives/aging_population/013988.html.

Weiten, W., Lloyd, M. A., Dunn, D. S., & Hammer, E. Y. (2009). *Psychology applied to modern life: Adjustment in the 21st century* (9th ed.). Pacific Grove, CA: Wadsworth/Cengage.

2

A History of Helping

It is important to know the path human services has taken to arrive at its present place in history in order to more fully understand human services today. Social welfare legislation, which has not only been an integral part of human services in the United States but also reflects the values of society, illustrates this path well. Tracing the historical development of human services provides answers to questions about changing human needs, emerging client groups, societal conditions, and responses to human need.

The chapter begins with an exercise that connects the content of Chapter 2 in *Introduction to Human Services, 7th ed.* to the cases and applications in this chapter. The second exercise encourages you to think about your ideas about welfare. It is followed by a list of important terms and their definitions. Next, a focus on American social welfare legislation prepares you for a case study of a welfare recipient. Answering the questions that follow and reading the perspective of a human service professional will add to your understanding of the welfare system.

INTRODUCTION

Review Chapter 2 in your textbook, *Introduction to Human Services, 7th ed.* Summarize human service delivery in U.S. history. Begin by listing what services were available during each of these four periods:

- Colonial America

_____

_____

_____

_____

- Civil War

_____

_____

_____

_____

_____

- Great Depression

_____

_____

_____

_____

_____

- The Great Society

_____

_____

_____

_____

_____

Describe the needs met by the services you listed above. Which needs are present across periods in history? Which needs reflect unique circumstances?

_____

_____

_____

_____

EXERCISE: WHAT ABOUT YOU?

Imagine that you are on welfare. Based on what you know about welfare today, what do you think your life would be like? Describe your housing, your food, your daily activities, and your family and friends. Next, identify the services that would be helpful to you. Why did you choose these services?

_____

_____

_____

_____

_____

_____

_____

KEY IDEAS

Human services have developed throughout history because there have always been people in need. Families with children (especially single mothers with children) who live in poverty have long been seen as potential clients who require assistance. The following terms provide an historical perspective concerning the history of services with special emphasis upon families and children.

The Church

Prior to the 1500s, the Catholic Church was the main provider of human services in Europe, founding institutions to serve the poor, the elderly, and those with disabilities. During the Middle Ages, generally accepted beliefs attributed most deviant behavior to a sickness, requiring the establishment of asylums.

Elizabethan Poor Laws of 1601

In England, these laws ensured that those in need received governmental help. The need for laws emerged as industrialization encouraged the development and growth of cities and the disintegration of the feudal estates, prompting the movement of the population from rural to urban areas. Untrained workers seeking employment in factories along with the disabled, widows, dependent children, the elderly, and individuals with mental problems, needed basic food, housing, and clothing. These laws were the model for human services in colonial America.

Child Welfare

From the mid-19th century to the beginning of the 20th century in the United States, the treatment of children in need changed. Many were removed from institutions that served all ages of the poor and placed in private homes. Orphanages were established for children without parental support. Homes that targeted individuals with special needs such as emotional disturbances and juvenile delinquency were established as well.

Federal Involvement

Throughout Western history, the involvement of the government in human services has waxed and waned. Following the decline of the Catholic Church as the primary human service provider during the Middle Ages in Europe, the role shifted to the government with the passage of the Elizabethan Poor Laws of 1601. Even in the United States, participation in human services has evolved, reaching its greatest expansion with the Social Security Act of 1935. This trend reversed during the 1980s, resulting in drastic cutbacks in the programs serving those in need and culminating in welfare reform during the 1990s. Today, questions about the necessity and efficacy of social services continue in the United States even during recession.

Aid to Families with Dependent Children (AFDC)

First established by the Social Security Act of 1935 as Aid to Dependent Children, this program provided public assistance to dependents and survivors of workers. Underlying this legislation and this program was the belief that the American people had a right to or were entitled to benefits. AFDC is the program that became generally known as "welfare" to the public.

Human Service Movement

In response to the emphasis upon developing human service programs during the 1960s, the demand increased for human service professionals to staff these programs. The Southern Regional Education Board (SREB), with the support of the National Institute for Mental Health (NIMH), developed educational programs to prepare entry-level professionals to provide direct services, especially to mentally ill clients. These new professionals were the forerunners of the thousands of helpers with associate and baccalaureate degrees who provide services in the fields of criminal justice, gerontology, child and adolescent services, family services, mental health, and many others.

Personal Responsibility and Work Opportunity Reconciliation Act (PRWORA)

Passed in 1996, this legislation abolished Aid to Families with Dependent Children (AFDC), one large public assistance program initially established as a part of the Social Security Act of 1935. Its passage reflected the change in attitude concerning social services that resulted in a reduction of federal and state monies allocated to social services, as well as a belief that aid programs provided to individuals should be more short term in duration. With the passage of PRWORA, the states also increased their role in program development and the allocation of funds. The purpose of PRWORA was twofold—to reduce the number of families on welfare and to encourage parents of young children to seek employment. The program was not developed to eradicate poverty.

Temporary Assistance for Needy Families (TANF)

This program was created by the Personal Responsibility and Work Opportunity Reconciliation Act (PRWORA) to replace the Aid to Families with Dependent Children (AFDC), Emergency Assistance (EA), and Basic Skills Training (JOBS). TANF gave states and territories the right to develop their own programs through block grants. The purposes of TANF include assisting needy families so that children can be cared for in their own homes; reducing the dependency of needy parents by promoting job preparation, work, and marriage; preventing out-of-wedlock pregnancies; and encouraging the formation and maintenance of two-parent families (Social Security Administration, 2009). According to TANF guidelines, each state must meet specific outcomes such as a designated percentage of families coming off assistance.

EXERCISE: YOU AND WELFARE

Reread your personal account of your life on welfare from the "What About You?" exercise. Assume that you have been receiving welfare payments for the past five years and that you are now moving out of the welfare system and into the workforce as dictated by the new welfare reform legislation. Describe the type of support you will need if you are to join the workforce. What will the barriers be? Will you be successful? Why or why not?

FOCUS: SOCIAL WELFARE LEGISLATION

One of the important ways that human needs have been met throughout the last few centuries is through social welfare legislation because this legislation reflects a society's values about meeting the needs of its people—what is important and how priorities are translated into action. Social welfare legislation itself represents a particular point of view about government and its responsibilities. For instance, within the context of social welfare legislation, the government both provides or purchases services and establishes rules by which those services are developed and distributed.

The foundations of social welfare in the United States are important to understand as we examine social welfare today. This section will highlight three examples of social welfare legislation that illustrate its development in the United States in response to society's changing needs and values.

It is important first to understand the role of government and legislation in meeting human needs. In the United States, the government often has been a provider of human services; this occurred through the legislative process. How did it come to be this way? As with many other societal institutions, the American colonists looked to England as a source of ideas and strategies to deal with social problems. So the American social welfare system has its roots in English law, specifically the Elizabethan Poor Law of 1601, which provided the framework for human services in the United States. A brief look at some of the important parts of the Elizabethan Poor Law will help you understand the foundation it provided to the American social welfare system.

In England, the Elizabethan Poor Law of 1601 brought together several earlier pieces of inconsistent legislation that addressed the needs of people (Trattner, 1999). It is important to note that poor relief did not originate with this law, but had been a concern for a long time. As a cohesive statute, this law provided a prototype for human services and influenced American social welfare in several important ways. First, the Elizabethan Poor Law enacted a classification system of those who were in need: the able bodied poor, the impotent poor, and dependent children. Many services today still attempt to classify or diagnose as a prerequisite to service delivery. Second, the Elizabethan Poor Law incorporated the principle of local responsibility; that is, service delivery, such as it was at the time, was to occur in the community with selected citizens serving as overseers of the poor and as collectors of revenue. This principle clearly placed social welfare in the hands of a civil authority and instituted the collection of taxes to support its endeavors. The significance of this second point lies in the shift of responsibility both for services and finances from the church to the government, a situation that exists today.

A final point is the designation of parents as legally liable for the support of children and grandchildren and children as legally responsible for parents and grandparents. If these designees could not provide for their needs, then human services became the responsibility of the government—the beginnings of a welfare bureaucracy. The term *welfare bureaucracy* is used quite often today to refer to the government's involvement in social welfare. The Elizabethan Poor Law was in effect for almost 250 years with only minor changes.

A second example of social welfare legislation that had profound effect on human services in the United States was the Social Security Act of 1935. It was a significant shift in meeting the needs of citizens for several reasons. Most importantly, this law was designed to provide security to protect individuals from unforeseen catastrophes. As part of President Franklin Delano Roosevelt's New Deal, the legislation responded to the economic depression that had devastated many individuals and families. By assisting in the maintenance of the financial well-being of those who were eligible, the Social Security Act ensured protection from economic instability. It also established a national system of welfare activities that improved the treatment of the poor, primarily because of the provision for cash payments to individuals in cases of unemployment, disability, and old age, thus preventing destitution.

Underlying this provision was the belief that the American people had a right to public benefits. No longer were social and economic problems viewed as the weakness of an individual. Finally, the Social Security Act added a new word to the social welfare vocabulary; the idea of *entitlements* as national policy meant that the federal government assumed responsibility for its citizens by making funds to finance this and other New Deal programs a part of the federal budget. This idea resulted in a new policy of federal aid to the states, ending more than 300 years of the poor law and its principle of local responsibility. Many consider the passing of the Social Security Act of 1935 to be the birth of the American welfare state.

What exactly was the Social Security Act? This landmark legislation provided for a federal program of old age retirement benefits and a joint federal-state venture of unemployment compensation. It also dispensed federal funds to states to develop such programs as vocational rehabilitation, public health services, and child welfare services, along with assistance to the elderly and the disabled. The Social Security Act also instituted a system of mandatory old-age insurance that based benefits on the previous earnings of persons over the age of 65 and established a reserve fund financed through the imposition of payroll taxes on employers and employees.

When the Act was passed, only employees in industrial and commercial occupations were eligible for protection. Since 1935, a number of amendments have expanded the categories of coverage. For example, in 1939, Old-Age Insurance began to serve families as dependents and survivors of workers were eligible for benefits. In 1950, coverage was expanded to jobs outside commerce and industry, including domestic and farm workers, employees of state and local governments, and employees of nonprofit organizations. In 1965, the Medicare program was added to include health insurance benefits for persons over the age of 65. Social Security programs continued to develop programs to meet additional needs. Those programs include school breakfasts; black lung benefits; supplemental security income; special supplemental food program for women, infants, and children; earned income tax credit; and low-income home energy assistance.

By the latter third of the 20th century, more and more Americans came to believe that the poor were to blame for their own circumstances. They also attributed part of the blame to the current welfare system because they believed it perpetuated cycles of dependency. In response to these changing beliefs, President Bill Clinton signed into law in August 1996 the Personal Responsibility and Work Opportunity Reconciliation Act (PRWORA), which effectively ended any national entitlement to welfare (Trattner, 1999). AFDC, the program commonly referred to as "welfare," was abolished, and replaced by a system of grants to the states that mandated the end of welfare to all recipients after two years, whether or not they had found jobs. The new program, Temporary Assistance for Needy Families (TANF), provides time-limited benefits that are closely tied to work requirements, which are intended to move welfare recipients off welfare and into the workforce (Institute for Research on Poverty, 2010).

Since 1996, the number of Americans dependent upon welfare has declined. National poverty data are calculated during the official U.S. Census using its definition of poverty. It is this definition that determines poverty by comparing pretax cash income with the poverty threshold which adjust for family size and composition. The threshold has remained fairly constant since its inception in 1966. In fact, the U.S. Census Bureau has revised its method of estimating the poverty threshold four times—in 1966, 1974, 1979, and 1981 (Institute for Research on Poverty, 2007). In 2008, the latest figures available at this writing reflect that 39.8 million people or 13.2 percent of the total U.S. population live in poverty.

Today, however, there is little consensus about the effects of welfare reform. Supporters cite declining caseloads, shrinking welfare bureaucracies, and more former welfare recipients working. Others suggest that only by looking at many other outcomes will there be an understanding of the true impact of welfare reform. These outcomes include changes in wages, employment and income, housing and homelessness, and levels of child maltreatment and foster care placement (Institute for Research on Poverty, 2007).

CASE STUDY: MEET JAMIE

The case that follows describes Jamie, who belongs to a third-generation welfare family. She is not presented as a typical or an atypical client. Rather, she provides us a view of the welfare reform of 1996 by sharing her story. She speaks in a rural American dialect, lives in an area with which many readers may be unfamiliar, and does not conform to many notions of the "good" client. As you read this case, focus on the challenges this client and her caseworker face implementing the new welfare legislation. Also try to identify any values or biases that you have about rural culture and noncompliant clients.

List of Characters

Jamie—young woman with five children who receives welfare

Momma—Jamie's mother; with whom Jamie and her children live

Will—Jamie's ex-husband and the father of all of her children

Ms. Bryant—Jamie's long-term welfare caseworker

Barry—Jamie's welfare-to-work case manager

Mr. Lewiston—Jamie's job coach

Part I: Welfare History

Jamie is participating in a welfare-to-work program. She lives in a rural area, and has lived in her family's house for most of her life. In fact, it was the house in which she was born. Her mother still lives there along with Jamie, Jamie's three children (her two other children are grown and have left the house), and other relatives who need a helping hand from time to time. At times, Jamie's two sisters and their families live in the house, too. The house is about five miles from town. Jamie's welfare caseworker, Ms. Bryant, lives in town. Sometimes Jamie considers Ms. Bryant her friend while occasionally, Jamie believes that Ms. Bryant does not like her at all. Jamie describes some of her welfare experiences below:

My granny was the first one in our family on welfare, and she raised up all of her young'uns that way. My momma was her second girl. They lived in the country about a mile from the school bus stop. In this house here. Momma talks about playin' hooky from school all the time. They'd start out fer the bus stop, and before you knowed it, all six of her brothers and sisters would be headin' in different directions, not fer the bus stop. My momma had three brothers who could raise all kinds of hell, so the school didn't worry much whether they went or not. Momma married at 14 and had six of us; she was on welfare the entire time and that was how we was raised. We lived with Granny, and none of us made it to school much. We just figured if school was important, then Momma would of made us go and whupped us good if we missed it. Why, she never did ask about school! That didn't mean that she didn't get into a peck of trouble fer it. The law come and got us ever' once in a while and took us to school, and Momma got called to the sheriff's office once about sendin' us to school.

But fer the most part, we was just too busy to get to school just roamin' those woods. That's how I met my ex-husband, Will. He was roamin' the woods too, and we usta roam together. He talked real nice and had strong hands, and one thing led to another, and we got married just before the baby was born. He was a wonderful daddy, but he weren't around much. I don't tell Ms. Bryant that he comes back to see us some. Did I tell you she's my caseworker? I think that she and I growed up together. Of course, she didn't have to walk to school, and she went regular like. She even went away fer a while, but then she came back. When I went on welfare, she was my worker.

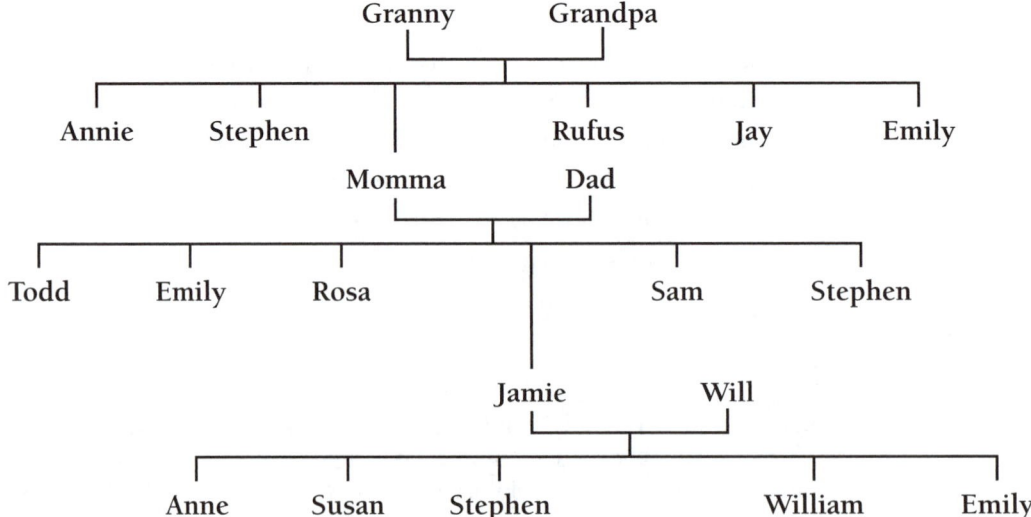

What a strange time that was, I wasn't a bit nervous about going to apply. Will and I had the baby and another comin' after we had been married nine months, and I hadn't never worked. Will couldn't find no job then. We needed money to take care of the baby and the one that was comin'. That was the only time that I lived away from my home. We rented a small house, but we couldn't afford to pay fer a phone and fer the electricity since we had the baby and neither one of us had a job.

Jamie used to go to the welfare office with her mother when she was little. So, when she had her first appointment there, she was somewhat familiar with the place. Her mother had told her that the caseworker would ask her a lot of questions, but Jamie was still amazed that there were so many questions. And she was not sure how to answer all of them. Jamie did know that it mattered how she answered the questions, since it would determine if she would receive support. She wanted to just tell Ms. Bryant that she was in the same shape as her Granny and her mother, but she knew that would not be smart.

Her mother had told her to tell the welfare office as little as possible. Jamie was warned not to tell about the money that she earned from Ms. Carlyle for babysitting her four children. She was also not to tell them about Will and how much she saw of him since he was in Kentucky looking for a job. So Jamie said that Will would try to send $10 a week if he had the money.

That first visit with the caseworker took over two hours. Ms. Bryant told Jamie that she would call her and let her know if she was able to receive the welfare services. Jamie left the office with confidence since her mother had helped her get ready for the interview. Here's what Jamie says about receiving the welfare support:

That's how my dealin's with Ms. Bryant started. I usta call her Miss Busby, and now that she's married, I call her Ms. Bryant. It seems like fer years I would go to see her ever' six months, and she'd ask me lots of questions. I'd answer in a way that would 'low me to get that check in the mailbox ever' month. Then ever'- thing seemed to change, all 'cept that I am still gettin' my checks.

I think that it started 'cause Ms. Bryant moved into that new building. Momma says that there's a new welfare law, and that's why there's a change. That's what Ms. Bryant says too, but I don't hold with it. See I reckon that they got to pay fer that new building, and they need to move some of us off welfare so they can pay fer it. Now the TV says that more people need to be off welfare, but it don't scare me. I know that I am gonna always get it. Let me tell you the reason why. But 'fore I do that maybe I had ought to tell you 'bout a visit I had with Ms. Bryant, the first time I went after they moved into that new building.

In the old building they was just gettin' started with their computers. I think that the welfare had started to change then. Granny used to talk about goin' to the food stamp office, which was the same place as the welfare office. Her and all her friends in town usta go at the same time; they had s'much fun seein' each other, and ever' once in a while one of 'em would make cookies to share. Well, they'd pick up their food stamps, bring their kids, and have what at church they would call a social. By the time they started gettin' the computers, it seemed to me that the social was long gone. Momma tells about those socials at the welfare office, but when she got growed, they weren't having them as much. But back to the computers. 'Member when I was tellin' you about the computers, and then all of the questions. All sudden-like Ms. Bryant didn't seem to have so much time fer me. She would ask me the same questions, and, of course she always asked about Will.

By this time we had four more kids, and we divorced. I told her that he only come back to see the kids 'bout once ever two months, but now that he had got a better job at the mine, he was sendin' me $15 a week. Really he was gone so much, and we wasn't married no more, so that wasn't a big lie. And me and the kids, we had us a great time ever' day. I spend all of my time with them. I hated to send them off to school, so I just send them off. They understand not to come home until about 2:00, just so I could say that they was gone.

Anyway, she usta to ask me the same questions, and then, she'd put what I'd say on the computer. It seemed to me that she was a mite frazzled, and she wasn't as glad to see me. She usta talk to me some about jobs; now she always talks with me about jobs and about trainin' and about education. My momma had always told me what to say, and what I said was really true. I didn't have time to work. And there ain't much work to be had around this town.

How do Jamie and her family survive with so little income? According to Jamie, the family does not have much money, so they do not spend much money. The house that they live in is about all that they have. And they believe they are lucky to have it. It has a bathroom, three bedrooms, a kitchen, and a living room with a fireplace. The fireplace keeps them warm during the winter months.

If something needs to be fixed in the house, then one of the boys or the husbands of one of the girls will do the repairs. Sometimes, they have to wait until they get equipment or tools to do the job. Just last spring the toilet in the bathroom broke and it took two months to get it fixed. The husband of Jamie's sister Rose had to wait until a toilet was removed from a house he was renovating before he could bring it home to install. They never throw anything away; instead they share with all members of the family.

The family is smart about clothes, too. All of the girls sew. And Jamie's mother can mend socks and shoes as well. They even have clothes to share with their neighbors. When Rosa, one of their neighbors, had her first baby last year, the family was able to pass down three blankets, two sleepers, and two little jumpers. Jamie says that the hand-me-downs that her children wear make them feel funny. They also are embarrassed about their haircuts. One Saturday a month, Jamie and her mother cut the children's hair on the back porch.

PART II: WELFARE REFORM

When the 1996 Welfare Reform Act was passed and the new Temporary Assistance for Needy Families (TANF) programs were put into place, Jamie's experience with welfare changed. She shares with us her initial impression of these changes:

Let me go back and tell you about the new welfare building and all of the changes. Not that I am too worried. In this new building there's even more computers than they was before. And Ms. Bryant only has 30 minutes to talk with me. It sure is different. She usta to be glad to see me, not that she ain't now, but she has to fill up her computer screen with the answers to her questions. She always has to okay my receivin' welfare, and now that I am pregnant again, we are puttin' in new stuff. Last time I was there, as I was leavin' I heard her call Will a "happy pappy." Momma didn't know what that meant, but my friend Jolene says that it means they believe that Will is sneakin' around and bein' with us more than we say he is. And that is suspicious since he's my ex. He comes to see the kids, and sometimes he comes to see me, too. Since I don't get out much, it's good to see him. Anyhow, Ms. Bryant says that these changes mean that I am now on a Families Forever State plan and that means that we have to do things different. I was powerful worried, but Momma says not to worry. There's always gonna be somebody to take care of us. It's just part of life. I trust Momma.

So we have to fill out this PRP. That's what Ms. Bryant calls it. At first I thought that she meant I had to sit in her chair and fill out the plan with her computer, but she had it printed up all nice. Fer the first time in a while she ask me what I wanted to do in the future. I told her stay at home and be with my kids and with the new baby that was comin'. She told me that by the laws I had to either go to school or get trainin' and then get me a job. Or I could go right to work. She was nice but kinda firm, not at all what I was used to. She also told me that I would have a case manager, somebody other than her, who would follow me around a bit and hep me get started with my new life. She also told me that I would have to be supportin' myself in two years, or I would be off welfare. I hate to tell you this, but I started laughin', well not laughin' but gigglin', you know how you do with your girlfriends. I could just imagine somebody followin' me 'round. Maybe they could hep with the house and the kids. Heavens, this person might enjoy roamin' the woods with the kids if she would come to visit. This new person was comin' to visit my home. Gracious!

I told her that I would have to think on this and could I come back, I needed to talk to Momma. I wasn't sure what to say and what to do, and I didn't wanna mess up, and I really didn't wanna to get pushed around. And Momma says that there's always a way 'round the rules. I headed back to see Momma as fast as I could. Ms. Bryant said I could come back next week. Momma, she really had the answers. She'd heard a little about this new welfare thing, but she couldn't figure it'd be coming here, we was just too small. So it throwed her off a little. She called her cousin in Chicago who knowed a little more about the new welfare plans they had there.

Accordin' to Cousin Lottie, who is on welfare and has lots of friends on welfare, ever'thing is changin'. Her welfare worker is makin' a big deal of these changes. She's gonna have to get her a job, go to school, make a plan, and learn to support herself. She knows that is impossible and really can't understand why her welfare worker don't understand that this plan won't work. Cousin Lottie ain't like me. Over the years she's had over ten welfare workers, some she likes, some like her; fer some she ain't got no use. You know what I mean. Anyway, she says that there's a ribbon cuttin' ceremony at her welfare office, and all of them on welfare are invited to come and hear speeches about what all is goin' on. She didn't go to the ceremony, but her friends that did go said that some of the talk was scary. Some of it was soundin' pretty good. But they all said the same thing: all them on welfare needs to be working in two years or they won't get no more money from the gov'ment. She even said that some of her friends were excited about the change because they'd have their own personal care helper work with them to find work and child care and they want some of them to be on a board where they can tell the government what to do. Chicago's a different place than here though. I can't even imagine where a body might work here abouts. Not that I wanna work.

Jamie returned to see Ms. Bryant, and Ms. Bryant provided her with a planning form that they needed to use to outline Jamie's welfare program. Ms. Bryant told Jamie about her new case manager, Barry, who would come to see her at home. The first visit was difficult for both Barry and Jamie. First, Barry had trouble finding the house. When he arrived, Jamie could tell that he was really nervous. He seemed to like the children but felt ill at ease sitting in the living room. His first responsibility was to conduct an interview; Jamie was frustrated because Ms. Bryant already had the answers to all of the questions in her files. He told her that he wanted to hear her story firsthand. Then, Barry explained the new program:

Then what he done surprised me. And it surprised Momma, too. She was there to make sure I didn't get myself into no trouble. He give me a list that had what he calls "options" on it about the things that I could do in the next two years. This page was plumb chock full of what he called opportunities, some didn't look too bad, but some of them just looked awful. The list we looked at had two columns, one was education and trainin' opportunities and the other was work opportunities—or so he said. It was clear to me that he didn't understand, so I asked him if he wanted soda or a glass of water. He was still nervous, just kinda looked 'round and said, "No thanks." Anyhow, he said that if I was to git my welfare check, that I had to choose one of them "opportunities" and be a "eager participant." He kept usin' that word. I hadn't never been called a participant before.

Momma told me that the more that I kept him talkin', the less harm, so she and I asked him to go over ever one of the "options" and tell us about 'em. Well, he done that. There was nothing that I could or would wanna do on the list. Why would I wanna change what I am doin' now? He said he'd leave the list with me, and he wanted to come back tomorrow and help me make a plan. I told him that I was busy, so he said he'd come the next day. I wanted to make him a cake, but I figured he didn't wanna eat from my kitchen. Well, I made him one just the same. I 'member when I was young like him. Did I tell you he looked a little like Michael Douglas? I didn't tell him so. Momma thought so, too.

I decided right then and there that I'd act like I was ready to make a plan. None of it looked good to me, but heck, this might be just like leavin' the house ever'day fer school and fer the bus, but never gettin' there. How can they think about takin' me off welfare? I need the money to take care of my kids. I forgot to tell you, he asked all sorts of questions about Will. He was all red and bashful when he asked. I think what he wanted to know, "Where is Will? He must come to visit since you keep getting pregnant all of the time?" I never did answer none of the questions. Momma said only use one sentence when I talk about Will. "He works the mines and we're divorced; he come to see the kids once ever two months fer two days, and he sends $15 dollars a month to help support the kids." I can say that sentence in my sleep, so I did.

Well, Barry he showed up the next day, and we did make a plan. Our town is changin' so much. Now we got us a red light in the middle of town, and we got a McDonald's. So our plan included six months trainin' at the local welfare and the McDonald's. And Barry was gonna hep me find somebody to look after the kids. That was a joke since I live so far out in the woods, but he said that he would hep me. I usta work only with Ms. Bryant, so all of this attention kinda made my head spin. Besides Barry, I had what they called a job coach, Mr. Lewiston from up in the western part of the state. I was supposed to go to class ever'day fer seven weeks. Can you imagine that? Never in my life did I go to class so much, and certainly not when I had all of these kids. It was gonna be hard!

Anyhow, some of the stuff that they was tryin' to teach us was interesting, things like how to apply fer a job and how to balance a checkbook. But then a checkbook is fer money in the bank, and I never did have no bank account. What little money I got is kept in three places. First, I got my own personal stash, and I ain't tellin' where that is, but I have $45 there. Then I've a jar under the mattress that I keep money just in case there's an emergency. I got $60 there. And I keep the rest in a cookie tin up on the top shelf of the cabinet. That's the rest of my welfare money. I use that fer groceries and gas and extra things fer the kids. Every kid that comes in my house knows where that money is, they also know that there's hell to pay if they was to touch it.

Jamie's new classes were very structured. She was taking English, math, and social studies. At the end of each instructional section, Jamie had to pass a test. Jamie and Barry signed a plan that stated she would go to classes at least four times a week. She managed to get to class about twice a week. If she missed two days in a row, then Barry would come by her house to find out why she missed class. He had trouble getting her by telephone since it does not always have a clear connection.

After a month of class work, Barry had a serious discussion with Jamie about her performance. Jamie just listened to Barry but did not talk very much. Her mother was not at home that day and Jamie was afraid that she would say the wrong thing to him. She was afraid to tell him that she could not make the child care work. Barry told her that welfare would provide money for child care, but the only care Jamie could find was with a woman who lived on the outskirts of town. After Barry left, Jamie vowed she would try harder to use the child care. For several days in a row, she rang the bell of the childcare worker, but no one even answered. She missed more classes, and Barry returned to see her:

So Barry come by all serious and said that he was disappointed in me: "You have not been attending your classes regularly and that means you are not following the plan you signed." I felt bad about it. Honest I did. Well at least at little bit, and I was tryin'. But when there's nowhere to take the kids, what do you want me to do? That is what I asked him. He said I shoulda called him and let him know. He also said that now I had done missed so many days, I would hafta start all over again. The new program started in three weeks, and I could start then. I could tell that he wanted to talk with me about changin' my life. He wanted me to work and set a good example fer my kids.

I listened, and he talked, and I smiled, and he thought that I agreed with him. He left happy. What he don't understand is I'm just as happy as I can be and my kids are, too. "Looka here," I wanted to say to him, "You ain't got no idea what you're talkin' about. Sure we ain't got big fancy houses and big cars, but we got a great family and we give our kids lots of time. That's more important than money." I loved the times that I was able to walk to the bus with my brothers and sisters and never did make it to school. It felt good just bein' in the woods. Momma says that we can live on the land, use welfare to pay our few bills, and not owe nobody nothin'. And of course, there's the money Will sends, and I'm not ever tellin' how much or how often he come to visit. That's just between me and Will and Momma.

I call what Barry and I do "dancin' in the dark." I really knowed he tries to hep me and he thinks he's got great big plans fer my life. After I had such poor attendance fer the first two programs, well, you know, first it's childcare problems, and then it's feeling poorly. And then, it's just not wantin' to go or just wantin' to go to visit one of the neighbors. So, he decided that I should change my plan.

But before that, Ms. Bryant called me in 'cause she wanted to talk with me. Momma went with me. She is protective, but she also wanted to know what Ms. Bryant had to say. Ms. Bryant, I could tell that she hated to tell me the news that she did. She said that she would have to report that I wasn't makin' no progress on my plan and that I wasn't cooperating. She was making notes on her computer when she was talkin' with me. She tried to be patient and kind, but even I could see she was kinda upset. She asked if I wanted a new case manager; she asked if I wanted to stay in the program. She told me I was in danger of losing my welfare, since my progress had to be reviewed ever' six months. This was the second report in a year that she had to make that said I was not doing what I was supposed to be doing.

Ms. Bryant said that I had one more year to be on welfare, and then I would hafta to get a job. Momma warned me not to get too uppity with Ms. Bryant so I just listened. She had knowed me fer such a long time; I'm a good mother; I love my kids; and I use my welfare check to support them. I do so well I don't even need food stamps, but I do use the state insurance. Didn't Ms. Bryant remember how she had heped me get that insurance? Now that's Barry's job, and he heps me fill out the form that lets me stay in it. She asked me why I had dropped out of the trainin' fer the third time and 'minded me that the best attendance that I had was comin' two out of ten times. Fer me that was really good. She asked if I wanted to get my GED. I asked her what was a GED. She told me that I'd be able to say that I had graduated high school. I never even wanted to graduate from junior high. I was quiet about that. She then told me that I'd wasted two years, and that she might not be able to keep my welfare fer the next year. I asked what she meant, but I knowed."

So Jamie told Ms. Bryant that she would go to work. She had the choices of three different fast food restaurants in the area. Jamie still had questions since she did not have access to good child care and she was never sure if her car would make it to town or not. But she held those comments to herself. Ms. Bryant told Jamie that Barry would come by with the papers to change the plans that they had made. Barry would be the one to confirm the job location.

That conversation with Ms. Bryant occurred three years ago. In those three years, Jamie has worked a total of four months. No matter how hard she tries, maintaining steady employment is difficult for her. Challenges such as child care, unreliable transportation, guilt over leaving her children alone after school, and evening and weekend work schedules, all made working very difficult and have contributed to Jamie's lack of motivation to work.

Jamie still has a case manager; in fact, she has had three of them since Barry. And she goes to see Ms. Bryant every three months now. Most of the time she goes without her mother. Jamie is not sure how long she will be able to stay on welfare, and she sees few alternatives for herself and her family.

Case Questions

1. Describe Granny and Momma's welfare history.

_____

_____

_____

_____

_____

_____

_____

_____

2. What were Granny and Momma's attitudes toward receiving welfare?

_____

_____

_____

_____

_____

_____

_____

_____

3. Describe Jamie's history of receiving welfare. How did the system change while she was a recipient? How did these changes affect her and her family?

_____

_____

_____

_____

_____

_____

_____

_____

4. Identify the positive contributions of the new welfare laws on Jamie's life and on the lives of her children.

_____

_____

_____

_____

_____

_____

_____

5. Identify the negative effects of the new welfare laws on Jamie's life and on the lives of her children.

_____

_____

_____

_____

_____

_____

_____

6. If Jamie were writing about the history of the welfare policy and its changing policies, what would she write?

_____

_____

_____

_____

_____

_____

_____

EXERCISE: YOU AS THE HUMAN SERVICE PROFESSIONAL

Now that you have an understanding of the history and present welfare policy and have read about Jamie and her family's involvement in the welfare programs, answer the following questions:

1. Describe your first reaction to any client who wants to remain on welfare.

_____

_____

_____

_____

_____

_____

_____

_____

2. Describe your reaction to Jamie and her situation.

_____

_____

_____

_____

_____

_____

_____

3. If you asked Jamie why she wanted to remain on welfare, what do you think she would tell you?

_____

_____

_____

_____

_____

_____

_____

_____

4. Barry worked with Jamie during a time of change in the welfare policy. What are the particular problems that he faced? How did he address them? Would you have handled the case as Barry did?

_____

_____

_____

_____

_____

_____

_____

5. If you were Ms. Bryant, would you continue to help Jamie? Why or why not?

_____

_____

_____

_____

_____

_____

_____

ANOTHER PERSPECTIVE: VAUGHN SMITH

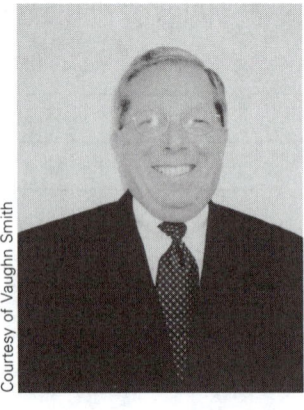

Courtesy of Vaughn Smith

Vaughn Smith is the director of the Work Force Connections program and part of the Community Action Committee (CAC) staff. The purpose of Work Force Connections is to develop and coordinate employment and training programs for welfare recipients. Vaughn assumes the responsibility for directing these employment and training programs, seeks new opportunities to provide services and solicit funding, and supervises the operation of the Career Center, Bridges Project, local Workforce Investment Act programs, and numerous state contracts related to welfare services. He holds a bachelor's degree in business administration and personnel management. Previous work experiences include job developer, counselor, and rehabilitation facility director at CAC. He has also served as Administrative Services Director for the Metropolitan Planning Commission.

Jamie has a number of values that are shared by the vast majority of Americans. She has strong family values and likes to spend time with her children. She is frugal, lives within her means, and is even able to share resources with other family members and neighbors. She has savings. Her primary concern is to feed and clothe her children, and she has figured out a way to do that to her satisfaction. Pursuit of happiness for herself and her family is her primary daily chore.

Unlike many other Americans, Jamie has no concept of self-sufficiency beyond welfare and sees no need to achieve it. She is a third-generation welfare recipient and has learned her values from her family just like the rest of us. She views others as living in a world that she will never see and never understand. But, she has managed to become content in the world that she understands. She has the support of her family, and her mother is a major influence and partner in her daily activities and the raising of her children.

The "system" or bureaucratic structure that allows Jamie and her family to survive is the local welfare system providing cash benefits and medical care. The members of this system do not attempt to understand why Jamie does not work and have little interest in understanding it. To use a metaphor, sometimes it is like "two ships passing in the night." Jamie lives her life on her own terms. Welfare exists in a separate world governed by its goals, rules, and regulations. Where the two worlds intersect, the focus is on providing welfare payments. The major activities in the system have more to do with determining eligibility than in promoting self-sufficiency. Hence, much of the interaction between Jamie and the system focuses on assessing criteria that determine if she is to receive services.

In this particular case I believe that the players in the system are either trying to reach the wrong goals or are clueless regarding how to work with Jamie. Poor Ms. Bryant is overburdened with paperwork (or computer work) and probably wonders what has become of her promising career in human services. Barry and Mr. Lewiston think that Jamie should suddenly become interested in pursuing self-sufficiency because the system "says" that she should. Many years of tolerance for welfare recipients has come to an end, and we expect the "participants" to completely rearrange their lives simply because we say so.

Working with Jamie: The Easy Part

To really help Jamie, services including transportation, child care, work readiness classes, GED preparation, and other services should be provided. The provision of these services is really a matter of money and logistics. Jamie points out the difficulty in obtaining reasonable child care for an evening job. Barry, however, left Jamie to arrange her own child care. Since this is a difficult task for Jamie, Barry needs to provide additional assistance in this area. Perhaps another family member can be paid to provide child care for the children needing it. Family-associated child care seems to be an arrangement that works, since work hours in fast food restaurants are primarily in the evening. Barry should suggest this alternative to Jamie, and if Jamie believes that this is a workable alternative, then he needs to help her arrange it. Transportation assistance should also be arranged in assisting Jamie to attend classes and work. Basic access to care often hinges on just "getting there" and transportation is a very basic service that must be provided. Jamie is uneducated and needs to develop basic skills. For this she simply must attend class. Hopefully, Barry can explore with her a way to attend courses, as well as GED classes, that work with her value system, her learning patterns, and will increase her interest in school. Simply providing classes for Jamie to take is not going to motivate her to attend. Some welfare mothers have begun to study with their children and that has motivated them to do well. Perhaps that approach will work in this case.

WORKING WITH JAMIE: THE HARD PART

Right now Jamie is interested in achieving and retaining eligibility to receive welfare. As long as eligibility is the focus, Jamie and the welfare system will focus on rules and regulations and not on Jamie's future. For Jamie to leave public assistance, she has to become interested in becoming self-sufficient. Activities leading to self-sufficiency should be the first priority on the list of things at which she spends her time and energy each day. This means that Jamie must change her system of personal values. She learned her values from birth from her family. New values can only be learned from experience. Short-term activities like job readiness classes cannot change the values acquired through years and generations of family training. How to achieve these changes is a major challenge for the system.

The community in which Jamie lives constitutes another difficult barrier. From the description in the case study, it appears to be fairly rural. Rural communities do not have an abundant supply of good jobs that pay a living wage. We keep poor people poor when we force them into fast food and other careers with no future. How can someone with three children at home be expected to live on wages from part-time, minimum-wage employment? No wonder Jamie has no interest in working. It will not improve her lifestyle and might negatively affect her welfare benefits. Why should we force Jamie to change her values, learn how to work, and join the workforce when there is no job for her with a self-sufficient wage?

CONCLUSION

Unfortunately, I believe that Jamie will never become self-sufficient. She will receive a variety of services; however, the barriers she must overcome are so formidable that she will never overcome them. Our under-funded systems are not adequate to solve all of her problems. We have no idea how to get Jamie to assume a new set of values that are more consistent with our own. She is smart and knows that we do not allow children in this country to be ill or hungry and that we will protect her while protecting them. Her benefits will end some day in the future when her children are adults. At that point, she will be dependent on her children to support her as best they can.

We must, however, continue to try. For each Jamie, there is someone on public assistance with fewer barriers. In communities where good jobs are plentiful, we have a much better chance at success. With many public assistance recipients, we can create the necessary value changes and they can be self-sufficient. We need more careers and career ladders that provide the opportunity for advancement in a short period of time. We need more subsidized child care and transportation for a longer period of time. We need a good system in which our recipients can learn a set of values that promotes self-sufficiency. We will continue to work toward these ends. It is important that we succeed.

EXERCISE: THE LAST WORD

You have the opportunity to have the last word on the terms introduced and the case study presented. Based on what you have learned in this chapter, answer the following questions.

1. When you think about what you have read about human services, what stands out for you?

_____

_____

_____

_____

_____

_____

2. How did the chapter change your ideas and understanding about human services?

_____

_____

_____

_____

_____

_____

3. How will you use the information in this chapter in your own life and work?

_____

_____

_____

_____

_____

_____

_____

4. What questions remain unanswered for you?

_____

_____

_____

_____

_____

_____

_____

FOR FURTHER STUDY

BOOKS

Ehrenreich, B. (2001). *Nickel and dimed: On (not) getting by in America: A life*. New York: Metropolitan/Owl/Holt. The author's three-month experience as an unskilled worker in Key West, Florida; Minneapolis; and Portland, Maine leads her to conclude that even for the worker holding two jobs, wages are too low and housing costs are too high.

Elshtain, J. B. (2002). *Jane Addams and the dream of American democracy*. New York: Basic. This book, based in large part on the writings of Jane Addams, portrays her as a pioneering social worker and a tough and visionary liberal.

Harrington, M. (1997). *The other America: Poverty in the United States*. New York: Scribner. Originally published in 1962, this classic account describes an isolated and self-perpetuating underclass that includes the elderly, children, and minorities.

FIRST-PERSON ACCOUNTS

Students may wish to read some primary sources that describe a particular historical period. The selections below represent first-person accounts of the late 1800s and early 1900s.

Addams, Jane. (1910). *Twenty years at Hull House*. New York: Macmillan.

Beers, Clifford. (1938 & 1939). *A mind that found itself*. Garden City, New York: Doubleday, Doran.

Brace, C. L. (1872). *The dangerous classes of New York and twenty years work among them*. Montclair, New Jersey: P. Smith.

Corner, George (Ed.). (1948). *The autobiography of Benjamin Rush*. Princeton, New Jersey: American Philosophical Society by Princeton University Press.

Richmond, Mary. (1969). *Friendly visiting among the poor*. New York: Macmillan.

Sanborn, Franklin. (1909). *Recollections of seventy years*. Boston: R. G. Badger.

Wald, Lillian. (1915). *The house on Henry Street*. New York: H. Holt.

MOVIES

A Home of Our Own (1993). Director: Tony Bill. Starring: Kathy Bates, Edward Furlong. Bates plays Frances Lacey, a single mother to six young children. Living in Los Angeles with nothing to predict a better future, she quits her job, packs her family in the car and leaves in search of a new home. In Idaho she finds the house that she wants for herself and her children. It is a shell of a house without a room, door, windows, or an outhouse. She mobilizes the family to rebuild this house so they can call it home.

Grapes of Wrath (1941). Director: John Ford. Starring: Henry Fonda, Jane Darwell, John Carradine, Ward Bond. This movie depicts the plight of individuals in depression-era America. It is adapted from the novel of the same name by John Steinbeck. The story begins in the Midwest where farmers, who were dispossessed, traveled to California to find work to support their families. The Joad family loaded their truck and left Oklahoma for California to be itinerant workers. Their struggle to leave Oklahoma, journey to California, and difficulties encountered in California all occur within the context of poverty. The movie illustrates the effects of poverty upon daily lives as well as long-term effects upon motivation and the human spirit.

WEB SITES

Explore the Web to learn more about the following:

Dorothea Dix	Bill Clinton
Hull House and Jane Addams	George W. Bush
The New Deal	Barack Obama
Social Security Act, 1935	AFDC
John F. Kennedy	poverty
Lyndon Johnson	PRWORA
Gerald Ford	social security act
Jimmy Carter	TANF
George H.W. Bush	welfare

REFERENCES

Institute for Research on Poverty. (2007). *Who is poor.* Retrieved from http://www.irp.wisc.edu/faqs.

Institute for Research on Poverty. (2010). *Economic stimulus and state TANF programs.* Retrieved from http://www.irp.wis.edu/dispatch/2010/02/22/economic-stimulus-and-state-tanf-programs/.

Social Security Administration. (2009). *Compilation of Social Security laws.* Retrieved from http://www.socialsecurity.gov/OP_Home/ssact/title04/0401.htm.

Trattner, Walter I. (1999). *From poor law to welfare state: A history of social welfare in America.* New York: The Free Press.

3   # HUMAN SERVICES TODAY

Like so many other organizations and institutions in society, several social, political, and economic realities impact human services. One way these realities are reflected is in how and where human services are delivered. This chapter explores the nature of human service delivery today as it is experienced by frontline human service professionals who know firsthand the daily challenges and future trends of their work.

The chapter begins with a short vignette that you can use to review the concepts learned in Chapter 3 of your textbook, *Introduction to Human Services, 7th ed*. A second exercise introduces you to a human service setting—a place where people can receive help—followed by a list of key concepts and their definitions. Then, a dialogue among five human service professionals explores their professional lives in five different human service settings. As you read about their work, you will learn about human services today in the United States. A human service professional then offers a perspective on this dialogue among the professionals followed by questions to consider as you develop your own understanding of human service delivery. Additional resources are listed for further exploration to conclude the chapter.

INTRODUCTION

The field of human services constantly changes and develops. Read the following short vignette, paying particular attention to human service trends as described in Chapter 3 of your textbook.

Sylvia Martinez is a helping professional in Miami, Florida. She is involved in resettling Cuban and Haitian immigrants in the United States. She is frustrated today because one immigrant family that she is expected to help cannot get the health care they need. They have signed up to receive care from an HMO in the northern part of the county but they have no transportation to the doctor's clinic. She is also frustrated because she usually provides short-term intervention; yet it will take weeks to resolve this medical dilemma. At the end of the day, Sylvia e-mails her supervisor to request additional time to work with this family.

List the ideas in the case that you believe are new to human services since 2000.

_____

_____

_____

_____

_____

EXERCISE: WHAT ABOUT YOU?

Interview an individual who provides human services. It may be someone in an office on your campus or a human service professional at a local agency. Describe the office or agency: its location, furniture and its arrangement, lighting and temperature, office equipment, and the manner and dress of staff. Focus your interview on the following topics:

*   Mission, structure, and funding of the agency
*   Recipients of services
*   Job responsibilities and titles of the staff
*   Motivations for choosing this work
*   Challenges for the staff
*   Trends or changes in the field

Summarize your interview here:

_____

_____

_____

_____

_____

_____

_____

_____

KEY IDEAS

The following terms relate to human service delivery both today and in the future. Their definitions will increase your understanding of the dialogue among the five human service professionals that follows.

CASE MANAGEMENT

This method of service delivery both coordinates and provides social services. Professionals who manage cases deliver help in a three-phase process of assessment, planning, and implementation that takes a client from intake to completion of the goal-oriented services and possible termination. Case management focuses on establishing a partnership with the client and other professionals that emphasizes integration of services.

COMMUNITY-BASED SERVICES

Providing human services to individuals, groups, or both on an outpatient basis in a community setting is a significant shift from the institutional-based services of the first half of the 20th century. This type of outreach impacted service delivery in several ways. First, sites of service delivery now include nontraditional settings such as schools, the military, religious organizations, and recreational facilities. Second, health and wellness are now part of the focus of treatment in community-based settings and third, case management, including clients and parents as case managers, is an accepted human service delivery methodology.

EMPLOYEE ASSISTANCE PROGRAMS (EAPs)

These programs offer services to employees of businesses and corporations to address the needs of their workers. These needs may include counseling for a variety of problems, wellness programs, and the development of work-related skills such as orientation, team building, and preparation for retirement.

SCHOOLS AS HUMAN SERVICE SETTINGS

Schools are one example of a nontraditional site for human service delivery. Often, schools and human service agencies share the same clients whose needs can be best met with a coordinated, collaborative partnership. This collaboration eliminates duplication of services, meets complex client needs, and maximizes resources. Working with children and youth with mental health issues within the context of the school is a way to offer integrated support services that melds quality education and human services.

MANAGED CARE

Managed care provides a way to control resources and deliver human services, especially in the areas of health care and mental health. Prior to the advent of managed care, agencies offered most services on a fee-for-service basis. Today managed care organizations control access to services, require increased documentation from service providers, emphasize case management as a method of delivering services, and promote resolution-focused assistance to limit the time and scope of services.

PRIVATIZATION

This term refers to the provision of social services by private companies and organizations. It signifies the move of service delivery from the public sector to the business sector and is predicated upon the belief that services can be provided from a business model, specifically, that profits can be made. Growth of businesses in the private sector includes prisons, hospitals, and mental health services.

CLIENT RESPONSIBILITY

This term refers to a change in the role of the client in human service delivery. For years the client was a passive recipient of services, accepting the decisions of others and following the direction of the helper. Today, with the emphasis on consumer satisfaction, client empowerment, and increased accountability, client responsibility has become a basic tenet of human service delivery. Clients are partners with helpers in human services by being actively engaged in the helping process, and by teaching helpers about themselves, their problems, and the services they need.

ADVOCACY

Speaking out on behalf of clients, especially for those who cannot speak for themselves, has become an increasingly important activity for the human service professional. It may involve empowering clients to act, improving environments, informing clients about opportunities, and guiding clients through changes and choices. On a larger scale, advocacy may mean informing the public, legislators, or both about needs or acting as a part of a collaborative effort in regard to a specific issue.

EXERCISE: YOU AND HUMAN SERVICES TODAY

This exercise will help you define your understanding of human services today in the United States. Before you answer the following questions, review the previous summary of your interview with a human service professional.

1. How does the term *community-based services* apply to the agency or office you visited?

_____

_____

_____

_____

_____

_____

_____

2. How does managed care affect service delivery in the agency?

_____

_____

_____

_____

_____

_____

_____

_____

3. Describe how the following might benefit clients at the agency you visited.
    Managed care

_____

_____

_____

_____

Client responsibility

_____

_____

_____

_____

Advocacy

_____

_____

_____

_____

Technology

_____

_____

_____

_____

FOCUS: HUMAN SERVICE AGENCIES AND ORGANIZATIONS

The most common arrangement for delivering human services in the United States is an agency or organization formed for the purpose of helping others. As such, it is the most typical setting for human service graduates as they begin their careers as human service professionals. Critical to successful employment and job performance in an agency is understanding the agency, who delivers services, what those services are, and to whom they are delivered. In the next section, you will first read a dialogue among a panel of five human service professionals. To increase your understanding of their perspectives as they discuss their jobs, agencies, clients, motivations, and challenges, you will read about the agency or organizational setting of human service delivery.

Many human service agencies and organizations exist to provide services to those in need. Services include education, health, mental health, criminal justice, and social welfare, as well as many others. They are found in both urban and rural areas of the country. To get a sense of the agencies in your area, check the yellow pages of the telephone directory under the heading *social services*. Many communities also publish directories that compile human service agencies alphabetically, by services, or by problems. You can also check the Web, Facebook, and Twitter for information about the array of services offered through the Internet. Some communities even have a telephone number similar to 911 that provides a referral for anyone who calls. These resources are also valuable to human service professionals who sometimes have difficulty keeping abreast of changes in agencies, services, and criteria for eligibility.

Human service agencies are commonly categorized by funding source such as nonprofit, public, and for-profit agencies. Private donations, fund-raisers, grants, and government contracts and grants fund nonprofit or voluntary agencies. Generally, a volunteer board of directors governs these types of agencies, and professionals, volunteers, or both staff them. Public agencies are a second category. Federal, state, regional, county, and city governments fund these agencies in order to provide services to a particular population. The funding source determines their operational rules and regulations.

Finally, a rapidly growing third category is for-profit agencies. They have two goals: (1) to provide a service and (2) to make a profit. Reduced funding of public agencies, the advent of managed care, and changing economic times necessitated the trend toward privatization and contributed to the growth in the number of for-profit, commercial, or private agencies in human services. Regardless of their funding source, one characteristic that all human service agencies and organizations have in common is a mission—usually a brief statement or summary of the goals of the agency and the population it serves. This statement provides information about its purpose and structure.

The human service professional is responsible for delivering services and is often considered a "frontline" practitioner. This individual works closely with the person seeking services from the initial request for services to termination. A job description, usually in writing, details the responsibilities of the human service professional within the context of the agency structure. Often job descriptions define the roles that a helper will fulfill. We explain these roles in more detail in Chapter 6. Unfortunately, a job description rarely reflects the actual work, although it does serve as a guideline. Many duties and responsibilities evolve given changing agency policies and procedures, client needs, and economic pressures.

A facet of human service delivery that can be both challenging and frustrating to the helper is change. The rapidity with which change occurs today exacerbates its effects on day-to-day work. Simply keeping track of trends in service delivery is challenging in and of itself. We highlight two trends here—the increasing use of technology and the prominence of managed care.

Technology is changing the nature of service delivery today. In fact, most agencies now use computers for information management, communication, and professional development. More creative applications of technology are evolving with the goal of providing human services more effectively and efficiently. The challenge for human service professionals is to maintain their skill level in order to use the available technology to benefit their clients.

Technology enhances communications among agency personnel, between agencies and the state or federal government, and between the client and human service professional. E-mail, teleconferencing, social networking, and the Web make available the most current information about client groups, helping strategies, resources, and research. Managing information and organizing and recording client data are also challenges.

Technology also impacts direct services to clients. Computer technology provides services that involve assessment, education, and counseling. The changes from technology are positive for the most part. Problems remain, however, and have not yet been overcome. These problems include the cost of technology, uniformity of services, and the confidentiality of client records.

Perhaps the most profound change in human service delivery in the past decade is the advent of managed care, and its movement into the areas of mental health care, child care, and corrections facilities continues to rise. How exactly has managed care impacted human service delivery? Direct services, which are the most affected, can offer several examples. First, service providers need different skills, particularly case management skills. In addition, managed care now emphasizes documentation for accountability purposes to meet both agency and managed care organization regulations. Gatekeepers control access to services and often propose resolution-focused or brief therapy as the preferred mode of treatment for short-term interventions. With this new structure for the provision of human services do come challenges. Managed care raises concerns about several issues, including the effectiveness of services that are limited in time and scope, the confidentiality of client information, and the quality of services amid budget-driven cuts in services and resources. Human service professionals must learn about the managed care system, work with such organizations to define practice standards, and contract with them for services.

CASE STUDY: MEET FIVE HUMAN SERVICE PROFESSIONALS

INTRODUCTION OF PANEL MEMBERS

Rachel Dove Peterson—is a therapist at a community mental health center. Her primary job responsibilities are group, individual, and family therapy; referrals and community resource linkage; crisis intervention; and assessments.

Her undergraduate degree is in human services and her master's degree is in social work. Previous work experience includes work at the Alzheimer's Association, a geriatric assessment program, and a psychiatric inpatient unit. For fun, Rachel enjoys her pets, boating, gardening, travel, and reading.

Bobby Fields, Jr.—works with Rachel at the community mental health center as a case manager. Much of his work is in the community as he helps clients with daily living needs, housing, problem solving, and transportation. He has also worked in an inpatient psychiatric setting for two years, but prefers being in the community with his clients. He has a bachelor's degree in psychology and enjoys singing, writing poetry and stories, and watching cartoons.

Stephanie Bailey—is a sign language interpreter whose primary responsibility is to facilitate communication between a deaf student and the teacher. She is an employee of the school system. Her academic background is in human services with a concentration in educational interpreting. She is married and has two young children. Her favorite sport is softball.

Kathy Wright—is regional director of the Arthritis Foundation, a position she has had for the past six years. In this position, she manages staff; provides information, programs, and services; and raises funds to support research. Previously, she was director of refugee resettlement for Catholic Charities in her community. She is a human service graduate. She and her husband raised five children and, as "empty nesters," now spend their free time hiking.

Jody Butler—is a counselor with an employee assistance program (EAP). Jody assesses client problems and provides short-term counseling, referral, and follow-up. She also conducts drug-free workplace workshops for companies. Jody has a master's degree in social work and is also a licensed alcohol and drug counselor. She has worked for ten years as an alcohol and drug counselor in both inpatient and outpatient facilities. Reading mysteries, swimming, and working in her flower garden provide relaxation.

PANEL DISCUSSION

DESCRIBE WHERE YOU WORK, YOUR RESPONSIBILITIES, AND YOUR CLIENTS.

RACHEL: I am currently employed at a mental health facility that serves children, adults, and the elderly. The program that I work with is a partial hospitalization program for adult patients who are part of the seriously persistently mentally ill (SPMI) population. These are people who have been in and out of psychiatric hospitals, on psychiatric medicines for some time, or both. We provide group therapy Monday through Friday—three groups a day. As a social worker, I lead two of them. One is led by a nurse. We bring these patients in when they are decompensating mentally and are at risk of going back into the hospital.

Our goal is to try to keep our clients living in the community. We monitor them on a daily basis. We have our own doctor who sees them at least once a week. It is a very successful program. People need extra time to be monitored and also to learn coping skills to deal with their mental illness. We see a lot of depression, anxiety, and some adjustment disorders. The program that I currently work with treats the adult population ages 18–55. We also have programs that treat the geriatric population who are over 55 years of age.

A limitation of this program is that it is only approved through Medicare. The majority of our patients at the mental health center are on a state managed-care program. So, there is this small group of people who are eligible for this program. If the patient doesn't have Medicare, we can't get paid to provide the service. That is one of the frustrations of the job.

BOBBY: I am a case manager at the mental health center. I go into the community to visit clients in their homes or wherever else they might be. My role is to make sure that they have the basic things they need—shelter, food, shopping. We do a lot of different things for them.

It is pretty interesting doing this type of work. I came from an inpatient program in the hospital to this outpatient program where I actually see clients in their homes where they are doing somewhat better. A lot of the homes that we see are not the best in the world. You can tell some clients live at the poverty level. I am there, though, and we talk about what is going on with them that day. Then, we set goals for what is going on in the future.

STEPHANIE: I am working at a middle school in the county as an educational interpreter. This means that I follow a deaf student who is being mainstreamed to each one of his classes. I facilitate communication between him and the teacher, or him and other students. One of the other services that I perform is to motivate him, provide encouragement, and get him to interact with the other children.

KATHY: I work for the Arthritis Foundation. I was a nontraditional student and I graduated in 1992. Besides having the pleasure of being in the human service program, I was able to attend class with a couple of my kids who were students at the same time. That was a special experience.

I have been with the Arthritis Foundation since I graduated. I started out as the director of the office here, fund-raising. I am now the director of this region, which includes 32 counties. I have three offices across the region with at least two staff members in each office. My agency is part of the National Arthritis Foundation.

In 1998, the Centers for Disease Control (CDC) and the National Public Health Department of the Arthritis Foundation wrote the National Arthritis Action Plan, because the CDC identified arthritis as the number-one cause of disability in this country. With the aging of America, the numbers of people who are going to have arthritis in the next 20 years is phenomenal. It's the number-one reason why people see their physicians in this country.

My role right now is to educate people about what they can do to prevent some of the complications from arthritis, and to reach out to the underserved in all of the counties in this region. To meet these responsibilities, I do a lot of collaborating. I work with the regional Office on Aging as well as with the many groups of people who service the elderly through programs throughout all of the counties. I actually have programs established in all of the counties. I work with all of the physicians in these areas, especially rheumatologists and orthopedic surgeons. Whenever a new person is diagnosed in a rheumatology office in this region, the staff suggests that they call my office to get more information. There are 100 different types of arthritis and we have literature on all of them.

The other thing that I do is to work with kids who have arthritis. A lot of kids have arthritis and we support their families in coming together to learn more about the disease.

JODY: I am working in an employee assistance program (EAP). I like this job because of the range of experiences I get. This EAP contracts with various companies in the area. So, the potential clientele of the EAP are employed. Actually, one of the employee benefits of working is access to the EAP. They or anyone in their household can get free counseling—up to

18 sessions a year. This includes marital counseling; counseling for their children, their family, or both; and for any depression or anxiety. These self-referrals are confidential, which means that nothing is reported to supervisors or employers. One of the things that I like is the extreme care in protecting people's confidentiality.

Supervisors can also refer an employee. The reason that they do this is to keep an employee. If the employee is having problems that are affecting job performance, and if the individual comes for counseling, assessment, or referral, then we can help this person keep the job and hopefully, make things better at the same time.

We also provide a lot of training with the companies. Drug-free workplace training allows employers to get a discount from the state on insurance—workman's compensation. We also provide training that is specifically requested, for example, sexual harassment, what to look for in employees who might be having alcohol or drug problems, or communication skills. The only bad thing about the training is that many of them occur at 6:00 A.M., when shifts are changing. Although I wouldn't want all 6:00 A.M. meetings, I enjoy them. You don't do just one thing all of the time; I am always learning. Even though six people might have depression or might have it to varying degrees, there are different causes, reasons, and goals. The treatment does not revolve around what I would want for them; it is what they want for themselves.

DESCRIBE YOUR CLIENTS—THEIR ENVIRONMENT, THEIR PROBLEMS, AND THEIR CHALLENGES.

RACHEL: We have people from every walk of life. Most patients who come to our program are low income. We've had people who have worked for 30 years, had some kind of tragic event, and now receive disability because their mental illness is so bad they cannot work any more. We have individuals who live in a group home or a boarding home. I have one lady now who has her own home that she rents with her three children. We have people who can drive themselves; we have people who can't.

Although we will take homeless individuals, we typically don't have much luck with homeless people just because we can't find them to get them to the center. We go to pick them up for the program and typically homeless people will either be in the shelter or out somewhere on the street. We don't have a lot of luck finding them unless they are very invested in care. We get people from time to time who want to get better, but who don't want to put the work toward getting better. They will come for a few days and decide that this is just a little too hard. It is easier to stay sick than it is to get better.

Getting better is a lot of hard work. You have to really try. You have to go home and do your homework that we give you in group. You have to really work on it. Those who don't want to work are not yet ready for the program. When they are ready, they will come complete the group, and learn. You can't force someone. If they don't have that drive to really work the program, they are not going to get a lot out of it.

BOBBY: I have 11 people on my caseload. A majority of them live in slum housing, the projects, or in some type of subsidized housing. A typical day for the client begins by waking up, taking medications, then staying home. Most of them have nothing to do. Some go out into the community with certain helping services, but the majority basically stays home. What is really interesting to me is that once I meet the individual, I can see the mental illness. Sometimes you meet the family and you understand more about the individual. I had one client who was on my caseload, and his mother was on someone else's caseload. In this family, there was mental illness in two generations.

STEPHANIE: Although I have worked with several types of students, currently the one that I have the most contact with has a lot of support from his family. The environment in which he lives is very wholesome—loving parents who are encouraging and active in his life. The goal is to provide support and encourage him to be successful in the mainstreaming program. He gets support from the hearing human service specialist, the interpreters, family, and the teachers. I think that this encouragement and support is vital for my deaf student's adjustment to the hearing world.

KATHY: Because arthritis is becoming such a major problem and because of the problems that we have in our medical system, far too often a person in his or her 50s or 60s will go to a physician and say, "I am having this problem." And the physician will say, "You know, it is part of the aging process. You have arthritis and there is nothing that you can do about it." That really isn't true. There are many things that you can do about it. Again, the people who are so underserved in so many of the outlying communities don't have this education and don't have the availability of the programs that we offer. That's what I am working on— to get into these communities.

    The incidence of arthritis is very high in this country—one out of every six individuals has arthritis. The latest statistic of incidence in our state is one out of three individuals. One reason is the lack of education. Another is people being overweight. It is a serious problem, and people think that they can just take a pill to make it go away.

    I have two types of clients. I have one group of people who never stop learning, get on the Web site, and have so much information that they call us every day and want to know about this new product. Then I have another group that goes home, sits in a chair, and doesn't move for two weeks because the doctor says that there is nothing to be done about it.

JODY: The clients referred by supervisors are often very angry—feeling like they have no control. Coming to see me is something that they had to do. Often they came in order to keep their job. They are often skeptical that I am really on their side. Sometimes that is a challenge. Sometimes the clients referred by supervisors are glad to have a mediator. They welcome somebody neutral and objective, a person who is able to see things from their side. It is really an easy clientele to work with because the self-referrals are there because they want to be. It is sometimes frustrating because they don't stay long enough to get all the help that I could provide. They get what they need and then quit coming.

WHAT IS THE GREATEST CHALLENGE YOU FACE IN YOUR WORK?

RACHEL: One problem that I have already mentioned is that there are so many people who could benefit from a partial hospitalization program, but we can only serve those with Medicare. That is very frustrating to me. When we had Medicare instead of the state managed care program, we used to have day treatment programs that could provide a lot of socialization, arts, and crafts. Now we have very strict guidelines, treatment plans, and objectives that we have to meet every day. If we cannot justify why a person is at the center and that they are working on something, we must discharge them. A therapist's view and Medicare's view oftentimes conflict. You know that person is improving and needs to stay longer, but you have to discharge him or her because we have got to have money to run the program, and we can't provide free services all of the time, although we do occasionally. That is probably the most frustrating thing for me.

BOBBY: The hardest thing about case management is a combination of two things. One is the lack of social support. There is no support from the family, friends, or associates. It is also the mind-set that "I'll never get better." Because of that mind-set, many clients sabotage their treatment. I've had a couple of instances where some have wanted to go into housing. They wanted to move out of their parents' home to live on their own. Once I get going, they are working toward this goal, and right before the client is ready to move in, he or she disap-pears. Clients might start using drugs again. They might fight or argue with family members and end up in jail. It seems like they don't want to succeed or they are scared to succeed. Success would take them away from what they know which is how to be sick and to feel sorry for themselves. They don't know how to get better. That is very frustrating.

STEPHANIE: One of the challenges that I deal with is making sure that the student understands what I am communicating to him, whether it is in math, science, or social studies. Depending on the subject matter, if he is not getting it, then I ask myself, "What do I do now? How do I simplify the information? How do I make him understand?" That is frustrating. Sometimes I need to tutor him after class or give him a good visual of what the instructor was trying to teach him.

KATHY: In my job I have two directions: fund-raising and educational programs and services. Obviously, my love is the educational programs and services, but I am also responsible for raising about $800,000 every year in order to pay for the programs and services and support research. That is part of the reason that the Arthritis Foundation exists.

I have so many other directions, too. Here is one example. We work a lot with kids who have arthritis. When kids get arthritis, it is a pretty serious disease, an autoimmune disease. The medications that they have to take are sometimes more harmful than the disease itself. You can't see arthritis in kids. Often, they are in the school system. Because they are kids, when they feel good, they do everything that everybody else does. When they feel bad, they can't do anything. If the school system isn't educated about arthritis, then we have problems.

For instance, a family might be reported for not getting a child to school on time on a regular basis because they have arthritis. When a child with arthritis gets up in the morning, it takes a longer time to get started. By 10:00 A.M., they are like every other kid again. By the end of the day, they may be dragging. We received a number of calls from parents asking for help with these school systems. School personnel didn't understand what it is like for children with arthritis. For a couple of years I worked with families on a one-on-one basis. Last year, I wrote a proposal for funding to do a workshop for school nurses in eight surrounding counties once a year. This one-day workshop explains the problems that kids have with arthritis. It explains how to identify it and what a teacher can expect in a student with arthritis. They simply didn't have this information.

JODY: To follow up Kathy's point, I worked with two children, ages 8 and 10, who were at risk for being placed in the state's custody because of truancy. They couldn't always get to school or would arrive late. The mother also had severe arthritis and fibromyalgia. Even though the school was trying to work with the children, they still had to follow the guidelines for days missed. It was very real and very scary for the mom to think that she could lose her kids because they were not going to school. I talked to Kathy about that last year, and she was very helpful.

The biggest challenge or concern I face in EAP is the time limit. Even though the benefit is 18 sessions in a year, we try to limit the sessions to 12, give or take a few, so that there are four to six sessions left in case there is a recurring crisis or if something comes up with another family member. Twelve sessions is not a lot. Basically what we can do is stabilize them, give them helpful advice, and try to refer them for longer-term care. It is hard to get them to follow through. Most people get to feel a little better and that is enough. The limit on number of sessions is challenging and frustrating.

WHAT ARE THE HIGHLIGHTS OF YOUR WORK—THE TIMES WHEN YOU ARE FEELING GOOD AND MOTIVATED TO CONTINUE IN HUMAN SERVICES?

RACHEL: One of the things that I like about working with people who are mentally ill is that the job is never, ever boring. I have worked in repetitive jobs before. No two people with schizophrenia are alike; no two people with depression are alike. The best therapist is a creative therapist who can approach a problem or situation from a different angle. To see people succeed is wonderful. We have a lady who has been in therapy on and off for years. She entered the program and said, "You know, I am really ready to do this. I am ready to change this time." We're real proud of her; she is doing great. You can have five or ten patients who don't succeed at all or don't succeed at such a high level, and you have that one who does. She makes it all worthwhile. Plus the people that you work with are really fun.

BOBBY: My greatest pleasure is actually seeing a change in someone. This may be reaching a goal, even a small goal. Here's an example. I had one client who did not bathe. In fact, he smelled pretty bad. The greatest accomplishment was when he came in one day and said, "Hey buddy, I took a bath last night!" He was happy about it; I was happy about it. Just seeing a client accomplish something is rewarding to me.

STEPHANIE: My greatest joy is seeing that my student has understood what I have communicated to him. He may think something is hard, but he will try. That means that he recognizes that it will be difficult for him, but is still willing to try. Hopefully, his efforts will prove to be successful and he will achieve his goals.

KATHY: What I like about my job is the variety. I do so many things. I have people who work for me, mostly young people, and I love teaching people about what I do. I really appreciate working with older people and giving them information that actually makes a difference in their lives. So many older people today exercise and swim. The Arthritis Foundation has a popular warm water aquatics class for people with arthritis. I was in a neighboring county recently to visit an aquatics class that celebrates every holiday by having a hat day in the pool. There were 53 adults in the pool with every form of hat that you can imagine—they were having a ball! These are people in their 60s and 70s. There are a lot of us in that age group now and life is changing for all of us. It is so nice to be a part of that opportunity for bigger and better things for them.

JODY: I like what I do because I enjoy seeing people feel better about themselves and their situation. They feel good and are able to handle things on their own. Even if they do need a little help, seeing people hopeful with a light in their eyes is what I like.

DESCRIBE THE ETHICAL DILEMMAS YOU ENCOUNTER IN YOUR WORK.

RACHEL: One of the biggest ethical dilemmas that I have encountered is suspecting abuse when you have a therapeutic relationship with a client. As a clinician it is your duty to report even suspicion of abuse. You want to do that for the child's sake. And you do report it knowing that it is probably going to completely blow the rapport you have with this client. You work so hard to know clients and help them. Sometimes you learn things that conflict with your ethics or your agency.

Another dilemma is confidentiality. I have worked with clients and I've thought, "If I could just talk to the parent(s), I could find out what is going on with this client." But the client is paranoid or doesn't like the parent(s), and won't sign a release so that I can talk to them. If a release isn't signed, it is the client's right to choose who you can talk to and who you can't. With no release, you can't get the information that you really want. Sometimes, that is hard.

BOBBY: I guess one of the hardest cases that I have ever had was a certain client who was living with his family. He was mentally ill. I wanted to get him into a group home or some type of home where he could get some help and begin to get better. But because he didn't want to move and the family didn't want him to move, he stayed with the family and didn't do too well. However, that was his choice. One of the hardest things to deal with on an outpatient basis is that clients have free will. They can do what they want to do; it is their choice. We have very little to say about it.

STEPHANIE: When a student is taking a test, I am facing the student. Of course, I am just looking at what he is marking. Facial expressions are very important in signing, and deaf people pick up on facial cues. I find it difficult to keep a straight face, especially if I see that the student is making a wrong answer. Now, I make it a point to move away to a different area of the room while testing is taking place. If he has a question, he raises his hand, and the teacher and I both go over. So, inadvertently giving an answer is an ethical dilemma I face in my occupation.

KATHY: We have a lot of support groups; the most popular support group is for patients with fibromyalgia. This is a syndrome that inflicts a lot of pain. Sleep patterns are disrupted. If you suffer from this disease long enough, you begin to have emotional problems as well. We don't actually lead support groups, but we train people how to lead them.

A big problem that we have is that there are many people selling treatments for arthritis that are not any good. They will contact these support groups saying, "We would like to be a guest speaker" with another guise or another reason why they are going to do this. I have actually been in a group where these people were planted in the audience. There were four people in this room of about 50 people who come for a support group for fibromyalgia. I began to realize after I was there for about 20 minutes that these people had a system. They were ready to put on a show for these people about this new cure. They want the group members to sign up immediately.

This is a real problem for older people. They get something in the mail every day about some magical, wonderful thing that is going to cure their arthritis. They are desperate for something to help so they are more than willing to try it. I always have to be alert to those who are going to take advantage of my situation and the situations of my clients. That is probably the biggest problem that I have.

JODY: A fine line to walk is often having a contract with an employer and a supervisory referral that enables us to work with the employee. Knowing what to chart and what to pass on is pretty scary because you have their livelihood in your hands. That can be difficult. Working with teenagers is also challenging. Rachel talked about building a relationship with them. You tell them up front that if they talk about safety issues such as suicide, drugs, or alcohol, you will have to involve their parents. They will tell you these things anyway. You have to decide how to work with them, so they will tell their parents. Making sure that they do and getting the parent involved without impairing that relationship is hard.

RACHEL, YOU TALKED ABOUT CLIENTS DOING HOMEWORK. WHAT KIND OF HOMEWORK IS IT AND WHAT WOULD THEY DO?

RACHEL: We do a lot of educational groups; for example, coping skills such as relaxation techniques and reframing your thoughts. If clients have these constant negative thoughts, we have a triple-column exercise that they can complete: what your thought was, what the situation was, and how you could reframe it in a positive way. We'll send exercises like that home with them and ask them to reframe two negative thoughts tonight and bring it in tomorrow. Another assignment is to practice one relaxation technique tonight that you have learned today. It could be deep breathing, taking a hot bath, or walking. This is a way for them to start doing it on their own. It's also a way to show us if they understand it or not, and if they have learned how to do it. Our program is limited to 30 days. It is real easy for clients to say that they are getting all of this, but if they don't practice it, then they won't use it when they are out of the program.

JODY, WHAT HAPPENS IF YOU HAVE A CLIENT WHO IS HAVING SOME KIND OF SUB-STANCE ABUSE PROBLEM AND AN EMPLOYER HAS SAID TO THE CLIENT, "YOU HAVE THIS PROBLEM AND YOU NEED HELP." WHAT IS THE PROCESS WHEN YOU DEAL WITH SUBSTANCE ABUSE?

JODY: The client is referred to us first. If a company has an EAP service, usually the employee is sent to an employee assistance counselor who does an assessment to see what the problem is and what level of care they might need. We try to match them with a facility that takes their insurance. We follow up treatment recommendations, and we coordinate with the client and the employer so that the employer knows that the client is doing what should be done about the problem.

IS THERE A GUARANTEE THAT THEY CAN RETURN TO THEIR EMPLOYMENT?

JODY: They usually know that up front. Some companies have a no-tolerance policy. Some companies will give an employee one chance. If the employee is doing what needs to be done, that is great. I have seen companies that will work with employees two or three times, but any more than that is usually detrimental.

WHY DID EACH OF YOU CHOOSE TO DO THE WORK THAT YOU DECIDED TO DO?

RACHEL: I was actually a business major and I don't know why. I think it was because I didn't know what else I wanted to do. I took a few classes and I hated it. I sat down with my mother and I said, "Mom, I hate this. I know this is what you do, but I really hate it." She said, "Rachel, I don't understand why you don't do what you enjoy." I looked at her and said, "What do I enjoy?" Obviously, she knew because she said, "You know, I have noticed that your favorite time of year is when we pick a needy child and buy them Christmas presents. You get totally into that. You love it." That was an interesting idea. I took the introductory human service course, and I knew that I was in the right place.

STEPHANIE: My story is pretty much like Rachel's. I was getting married and going to school part time. The plan was that after I got married, I would go full time. At the time I was in accounting which I didn't like. I could do the work, but I didn't want to be doing it for the rest of my life. My husband-to-be said, "Think about it and pick something that you enjoy because we all need to be in a profession that we enjoy." After some serious soul-searching, I remembered my interest in sign language. I talked to several people, and they directed me to the university to talk to one of the sign language instructors. We discussed a number of options but the one that fit me was human services with an interpreting component. I'm glad that I made that choice.

BOBBY: I will be honest. It was not the money. You don't choose this field to get rich. When I first came to college, I was going to be a business major. After I signed up I thought about it. I really don't have a business mind. I really like to help people. The day I signed up for my major I looked around and discovered psychology. I have always been interested in helping people and finding out why people do what they do.

KATHY: My story is a little bit different. I've been in human services all of my life. I have five children. Mary, my oldest child, was severely mentally retarded. She passed away two years ago at age 32. She lived at home until she was 24. During that time I was involved in every kind of organization, including getting a facility built for young adults who were severely retarded. Mary didn't walk, she didn't talk, and she lived at home until she was 24. When she left home, my life didn't fit any more. I just needed to do something different.

Actually, I started taking classes at the university so that I didn't have to talk to anybody. I could come to campus, spend the day here, and not relate to people. I was still very involved in lots of boards, schools, and activities. I happened to fall into the human service major and absolutely loved it. It has been an interesting and amazing experience. I had the wonderful luxury of being a stay-at-home-mom, raising five children, and doing all of the things that mothers can do. Then, I had the wonderful luxury of having a really nice job that I love. I am 57 years old and most of my peers are retiring, but I love what I do.

JODY: Actually, this field chose me. My life experience led me to work in a treatment center in the kitchen and housekeeping areas. I did that for almost a year when the director came downstairs and said that I was going to start counseling in a week or two. I told them that they were crazy. They won that argument. I started the training and working toward my state licensure and decided that I wanted to go back to school to get even more experience. The field placements opened my eyes to all of the possibilities and the opportunities to do any number of things with people.

THERE ARE LIMITATIONS TO WHAT EACH PROFESSIONAL CAN DO. WHEN YOU REACH THOSE LIMITATIONS WHAT DO YOU DO? DO YOU REFER? FIND OTHER SERVICES? DOES THE CLIENT GO WITHOUT?

RACHEL: What makes a good helping professional is someone who can utilize resources, network, and know what is available. I have a service directory that I use often. The best service out there right now is 211. It's a referral help line. I often call about specific services a client needs. As long as you stay on your toes, there is usually a service available. Sometimes there isn't. Transportation is the hardest. It's very difficult if you don't live on the bus line. Without transportation there is limited assistance unless you live on a bus line.

KATHY: I think this panel is a perfect example in that we all bring something to the table for each other. I deal with people with arthritis; they also have fibromyalgia and they have school problems. One of the greatest gifts that you have is that you have contact with other professionals. You cannot take care of everybody. That is the biggest problem in this job—burnout. If you think that you can change the world by fixing it, you can't. You have the resources of all your peers and everybody has something to offer.

CASE QUESTIONS

1. Describe the career paths of the panel members. List the different motivations that led each to pursue a career in human services.

   _____

   _____

   _____

   _____

   _____

   _____

   _____

   _____

2. Describe the current job responsibilities of a panel member. What does this person actually do in the course of a day at work?

_____

_____

_____

_____

_____

_____

_____

_____

3. What did you learn about each agency?

_____

_____

_____

_____

_____

_____

_____

_____

4. Describe how these agencies illustrate community-based services.

_____

_____

_____

_____

_____

_____

_____

5. What is the impact of managed care on the services provided by panel members?

_____

_____

_____

_____

_____

_____

_____

_____

6. Which panel member best illustrates advocacy? Explain your choice.

_____

_____

_____

_____

_____

_____

_____

7. How do panel members promote client responsibility?

_____

_____

_____

_____

_____

_____

8. Identify the nontraditional human service settings represented by the panel.

_____

_____

_____

_____

_____

_____

_____

9. Describe the challenges faced by each panel member in his or her daily
    work.

_____

_____

_____

_____

_____

_____

_____

10. What rewards make the work of these professionals worthwhile?

_____

_____

_____

_____

_____

_____

EXERCISE: YOU AS THE HUMAN SERVICE PROFESSIONAL

Now that you have an understanding of some of the basic human service terms
that describe human services today and have read about the work of five human
service professionals, answer the following questions:

1. What is your reaction to this panel?

_____

_____

_____

_____

_____

_____

_____

_____

2. Which of these jobs would you like to have? Why?

_____

_____

_____

_____

_____

_____

_____

_____

3. Choose two panel members and describe how you would deal with the challenges they face in their jobs.

_____

_____

_____

_____

_____

_____

_____

_____

4. Which client group would you like to work with? Why?

_____

_____

_____

_____

_____

_____

_____

_____

5. What qualities or characteristics do you have that would help you work effectively in an agency setting?

_____

_____

_____

_____

_____

_____

_____

6. What would be difficult for you?

_____

_____

_____

_____

_____

_____

_____

_____

ANOTHER PERSPECTIVE: PAUL ZAMBRANO

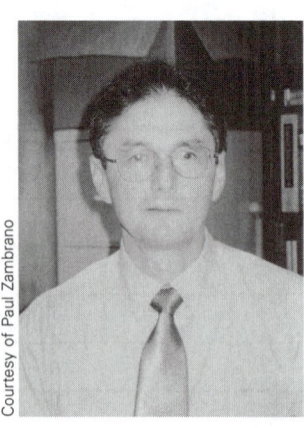

Courtesy of Paul Zambrano

Paul Zambrano, a case management supervisor, works with a culturally diverse staff of eight full-time case managers who provide services to over 400 individuals with HIV and AIDS. His job responsibilities include intake, case assignment, participation on a clinical team, staff supervision, and maintenance of the agency database. Paul has worked in several positions in human service agencies: director of a central intake unit, coordinator of outpatient mental health services, and coordinator of prevention and early intervention.

Paul's varied educational background includes an undergraduate degree in music with a concentration in theory and practice and graduate study in applied music at a university in Berlin, Germany. He also has a master's degree in counseling with an emphasis on agency counseling and family therapy.

I am left with two distinct overall impressions of the five human service professionals. First of all, I found it encouraging that they all demonstrated a high degree of awareness of what was important to them in life and how this was expressed in their jobs. This is a fundamentally important, yet sometimes overlooked aspect of career selection and personal development that will have profound effect on how service is provided. The level of self-knowledge displayed by the professionals and the resulting commitment to the profession is impressive. Secondly, and perhaps more obviously, was the great disparity in not only the job settings, but also in the ranges of responsibility. The greatest contrast in my view, was between Stephanie, the educational translator, whose sole focus was on finding ways of helping one handicapped pupil understand educational information (not an insignificant achievement, just narrow in scope); and Kathy, the regional director of the Arthritis Foundation who, in addition to supervision of staff, did large-scale fundraising, education, advocacy, and networking.

The two who were closest, at least in terms of the clientele that they served, were Rachel, the social worker, and Bobby, the case manager. They both served the seriously persistently mentally ill population. They were both realistic about the challenges of their jobs. Rachel demonstrated the ability to weather the frustrations of the situation, especially since she characterized the job as "never, ever boring" and "to see people succeed is wonderful." Bobby shared some of the difficulties he encounters as well as opportunities to work with clients in their homes.

Both Rachel and Bobby are now dealing with a chronic population for whom the probability of significant change seems minimal. Some frustration is to be expected and is evident in his statement that "the hardest thing to deal with ... is that clients have free will.... We have very little to say about it." Clearly, the effective use of free will is exactly what we should be trying to promote, but it is difficult to strike the balance between remaining expectantly hopeful that change will occur and feeling that we should dictate the speed and nature of that change.

The issue for several panel participants is how to focus on helping clients change. Bobby asserts that some clients "don't want to succeed or they are scared to succeed.... They don't know how to get better." He is likely correct in assessing the behavior and presentation of the clients. Even Kathy, the Regional Director of the Arthritis Foundation, talks about "two types of client ... one[s] ... who never stop learning ... and another ... that goes home, sits in a chair, and doesn't move." Our task is to try to determine what it is that we can do to bring this type of client closer to being able to take some initial steps toward changing maladaptive behaviors.

Many professionals struggle with determining just how much client participation is necessary to establish any kind of productive working relationship. This introduces a lot of gray area into the concept of client responsibility introduced under "Key Ideas" at the beginning of the chapter. The old adage that "If the professional is working harder than the client, something is wrong" is basically true since it is easy to create dependencies that can reinforce client's feelings of incompetence. However, low-functioning clients or clients with poor life skills are often unable to follow through according to our initial expectations. This creates the dilemma of either taking actions on the client's behalf that may enable the client to remain passive and unchanging or creating tension in the relationship by showing our disappointment when they do not follow through on expected actions.

Therefore, an absolutely essential skill for any practitioner is the accurate assessment of the present capacity of the client to change and the establishment of realistic goals to align with the present level of functioning. Initial steps in this process need not be dramatic or even very obvious. A simple internal change in a client's self-awareness is usually a necessary first step toward achieving observable behavior change. Two of the greatest dangers in this process are first, the under- or overestimation (especially over the long term), of what a client might achieve and second, imposing our judgment on what this means to the client. It is interesting that the professional with the ostensibly highest functioning clients (Jody, the EAP counselor) complains, "They don't stay long enough to get all the help that I could provide. They get what they need and then quit coming." Sometimes if clients get what they need, we have succeeded!

In my experience, another sometimes troublesome factor in working with clients who are not ready to change is the tendency of third-party individuals or other service providers to create unrealistically high expectations for the professional instead of for the client. These are people who generally take everything the client says, including complaints about the helper, at face value without checking with current service providers to ascertain the veracity or context of the assertions. The anxiety generated in the third party by the client's often exaggerated or partially accurate report of woe can be transferred to the primary helping professional in the form of a suggestion, or sometimes a complaint, or even a directive that we should really be doing more to help. This kind of misguided empathy can have crippling effects on a person's ability to change and grow and can actually perpetuate the very failures and inadequacies it was meant to relieve.

Agencies themselves can also collude to perpetuate client need since funding is often tied to numbers of clients served, which makes it desirable from a financial perspective, to retain contact over long periods of time. Capitated managed-care contracts that specify a maximum dollar amount for serving a given population are designed to remove the incentive to maintain long-term contact; however, providers often find that this limits their ability to deliver adequate service to the most needy. We must remember that the managed-care movement arose out of a situation where there were few controls, limits, or systems of accountability imposed on service delivery. Even though this can be a rather blunt instrument to adequately address the issue, some response was required to control spiraling costs and the tendency to promote dependency.

The overarching objective of being a human service provider is being attuned to the clients' processes of change, growth, and development on the micro and macro levels. We easily accept this idea in relation to the clients we serve, but the principle is also operative in our own lives and in the functioning of agencies and societal institutions. The shifting and interaction of these larger forces and attitudes will impact the culture in which we function, producing ever-changing work environments. Keeping the focus on where the client is in the process of change while enhancing awareness of our own processes will allow us to stay on track in what can be a simultaneously frustrating, yet exhilarating and rewarding, profession.

EXERCISE: THE LAST WORD

You have the opportunity to have the last word on the terms introduced and the case study presented. Based on what you have learned in this chapter, answer the following questions.

1. When you think about what you have read about human services, what stands out for you?

_____

_____

_____

_____

_____

_____

_____

2. How did the chapter change your ideas and understanding about what human services is?

_____

_____

_____

_____

_____

_____

_____

_____

3. How will you use the information in this chapter in your own life and work?

_____

_____

_____

_____

_____

_____

_____

4. What questions remain unanswered for you?

_____

_____

_____

_____

_____

_____

_____

_____

FOR FURTHER STUDY

BOOKS/PERIODICALS

Arthritis Today. This periodical by the Arthritis Foundation covers issues such as current research, nutrition, medication, exercise, and daily living products that make living with arthritis easier.

Corey, M., & Corey, G. (2006). *Becoming a helper*. Pacific Grove, California: Brooks Cole/Cengage. This text provides the reader with information about choosing to become a helper, the concerns of helpers, understanding diversity, and the process of self reflection.

Fearing, J. (2000). *Workplace intervention*. New York: Hazelden. This book describes the cost of addiction in the workplace and the ways to identify addictive behaviors, introduces interventions, expands the role of employee assistance programs, and explores legal, family, and violence issues.

Nathan, P., & Gorman, J. (Eds.). (2002). *A guide to treatments that work*. London: Oxford. This book describes in detail mental health interventions that work successfully with depression, anxiety disorders, and other mental health diagnoses.

Tehrani, N. (2004). *Workplace trauma: Concepts, assessments, and intervention*. New York: Brunner Routledge. The author explores the history of post-traumatic stress disorder, what trauma looks like in the workplace, and ways to anticipate, assess, and intervene to prevent and to response to crises.

Winston, E. A. (2005). *Educational interpreting: How it can succeed*. Chicago: University of Chicago Press. The author explores the profession of education interpreting and details the school setting in which it occurs.

MOVIES

In the three movies listed below, human service professionals, specifically counselors, play a prominent role.

Prime (2005). Director: Ben Younger. Starring: Meryl Streep, Uma Thurman. The movie depicts Dr. Lisa Metzger (Meryl Streep) as a therapist of Rafi Gardet (Uma Thurman), a 37-year old professional who has difficulty with relationships. The difficulties emerge when Rafi begins to date Dr. Metzger's son.

Good Will Hunting (1997). Director: Gus Van Sant. Starring: Matt Damon, Robin Williams. This is the story of a 20-year-old gifted mathematician (Matt Damon) who works as a janitor at MIT. He has had a difficult childhood and leads a very "rough" life. His gift is discovered by an MIT professor who employs Sean Maguire (Robin Williams) to counsel the young man to keep him out of jail and to encourage him to accept his giftedness.

Ordinary People (1980). Director: Robert Redford. Starring: Timothy Hutton, Donald Sutherland, Mary Tyler Moore, Judd Hirsch. The screenplay for this movie was based on a novel by Judith Guest. The plot revolved around Beth (Moore) and Calvin (Sutherland) as they try to recover from the death of their older son. Their younger son, Conrad (Hutton), experiences grief and guilt over the death of his older brother. He has attempted suicide and is in therapy with a psychologist (Hirsch). The dramatic tension focuses on Conrad's attempt to deal with his emotions, his mother's preference for her eldest son, and his father's role as the peacemaker.

WEB SITES

Explore the Web to learn more about the following:

National Organization for Human Services (home page)

National Organization for Human Services (home page and description of human service worker)

Arthritis Foundation

Employee Assistance Professionals Association

American Counseling Association

Educational Interpreting

advocacy

arthritis

community-based services

community mental health

employee assistance programs

managed care

Models of Human Service Delivery

A survey of the array of social services reveals variations on how services are delivered. The differences represent diversity in describing the problem, defining clients and helpers, establishing the goals of services, determining where and when treatment occurs, and determining method of treatment. Within this diversity of delivery, specific models or consistent ways of providing services have evolved in the United States. This chapter examines three prominent models of service delivery: medical, public health, and human services. While each model has its own distinct philosophy and history, all three make valuable contributions to appropriate, effective service delivery as they address client problems in life and work. Working together, professionals from each model facilitate change more effectively than any of the models working alone.

This chapter begins with an exercise that builds upon the concepts covered in Chapter 4 of *Introduction to Human Services, 7th ed*. The second exercise introduces you to the focus of this chapter—emergency and disaster services, and the application of models of service delivery. You will read about the nature of natural disasters such as tornadoes, hurricanes, and earthquakes and learn more about Hurricane Helena and the devastation it caused to those who lived through this storm. In addition, two representatives from the American Red Cross present another view of the hurricane and the emergency aid provided to the community. You will have the final word as you discuss what you have learned in this chapter and what questions remain for you. Additional resources for further exploration conclude the chapter.

INTRODUCTION

Read today's newspaper for your city or town. Based on the articles in today's edition, list the problems you believe are currently receiving the attention of the helping professions. Choose one problem and discuss how each model might address the problem.

_____

_____

_____

_____

_____

Based upon your understanding of these models after reading Chapter 4 in *Introduction to Human Services, 7th ed.*, what conclusions might you make about the strengths and weaknesses of each model?

_____

_____

_____

_____

_____

EXERCISE: WHAT ABOUT YOU?

Have you ever needed emergency services or been involved in a disaster? What about your family or friends? If so, describe your experience (or the experience of others) with emergency services or a disaster recovery service. Be sure to include the nature of the situation, the problem, the individuals involved, the services received, and the resolution.

_____

_____

_____

_____

_____

_____

_____

KEY IDEAS

Social services are provided using one or more models of service delivery. The three major models in this chapter have a distinctive focus and methods of treatment, and address different areas of human needs.

Medical Model

This model of service delivery provides help using an approach of symptom-diagnosis-treatment-cure. Traditionally, those who are helped are called *patients* and service providers are members of the healthcare professions. Patients are treated in an office or hospital setting, with a treatment goal of returning the individual to his or her prior state of health. The medical model has a long history that extends as far back as the Middle Ages when trephining (the removal of a circular area of skull bone), shamans, and witches treated mental illness. Today, the medical model is used to address the mental health needs of patients; psychiatric medications provide the foundation of the treatment. The strength of this model is a clear definition of the problem and the treatment goal. Its weakness lies in the prominence of the helper as the expert with minimal consideration of the patient's environment.

Public Health Model

The foundation of public health resides in the belief that the opportunity for good health is a basic human right. Those who work within the public health sector commit to examine the conditions in which people live, especially those in poverty, and to improve their conditions. The public health model bridges the medical and the human service models as it focuses on education, nutrition, safe food and water, immunization, and maternal and child health. According to the definitions of this model, the clients represent individuals and special populations or geographic areas. Helpers combine medical knowledge with community action skills to address problems and to try to prevent them. The strength of this model is its focus on prevention and its commitment to improve the lives of the poor. The weakness is its attention to the community that, at times, ignores individual needs.

Human Service Model

Within the framework of the human service model, helpers from a variety of professions address internal, environmental, and intrapersonal problems in living described in Chapter 1. Clients are defined as individuals, families, special populations, and environments. The problem-solving process is the method of treatment. Using this process, helpers and clients partner to address client needs by focusing on strengths, resources, and resilience. Human service professionals recognize that most clients have more than one problem. An interdisciplinary approach provides the most effective care to address these multiple issues. This approach involves several professionals in the helping process and increases the clients' chances for growth. The strength of this model is the involvement of the client as a participant in the helping process, as well as teaching the client to use the problem-solving process. The weakness of this model is the difficulty in focusing on one issue or setting clear goals.

EXERCISE: YOU AND SERVICE DELIVERY MODELS

This exercise will help you think about models of service delivery in light of your own experiences. Before you answer these questions, review your response to the "What About You?" exercise at the beginning of the chapter.

1. In the emergency or disaster situation that you described earlier in the chapter, identify the services you (or others) received that reflect the medical model. Explain.

   _____

   _____

   _____

   _____

   _____

   _____

   _____

   _____

2. In the emergency or disaster situation that you (or others) described earlier in the chapter, identify the services you received that reflect the public health model. Explain.

   _____

   _____

   _____

   _____

   _____

   _____

   _____

   _____

3. In the emergency or disaster situation that you (or others) described earlier in the chapter, identify the services you received that reflect the human service model. Explain.

   _____

   _____

   _____

   _____

   _____

   _____

   _____

TABLE 4.1 | AN OVERVIEW OF THREE MODELS OF SERVICE DELIVERY

	View of the problem client?	Who is the client?	Who is the helper?	Where does Treatment occur?	Method of treatment	Goal of Treatment
Medical	Individual has a physiologically based illness or disease	Individual who receives services is called a patient	Trained professional in health sciences (physician, nurse, dentist, psychiatrist)	Office Institution	Diagnosis Treatment Behavioral prescription Medication Psychoanalysis	Return individual to prior state
Public Health	Individual, groups, and society have disease or illness Environmental and social pressures also contribute to problem	Individuals and special populations or geographic areas (community, neighborhood, state, nation) can be clients	Public health training combines medical knowledge with community action skills	Office Community	Medical diagnosis Prescription Education Mobilization of resources Advocacy for special populations	Prevention Social action
Human Services	"Problems in living" may be internal, environmental, and/or intrapersonal	Individuals, families, special populations, and environment can be clients	Volunteer Paraprofessional Entry-level human helper who works with abuse, rehabilitation, education, etc. Professionals (rehabilitation or mental health counselor, social worker, psychologist)	Offices/ agencies/ institutions serving individuals, families, children Community	Problem-solving process Strengths identification	Enhance client's well-being, and quality of life Teach client problem-solving skills Prevention

FOCUS: EMERGENCY AND DISASTER SERVICES

"Disaster. It strikes anytime, anywhere. It takes many forms—a hurricane, an earthquake, a tornado, a flood, a fire or a hazardous spill, an act of nature or an act of terrorism. It builds over days or weeks, or hits suddenly, without warning. Every year, millions of Americans face disaster, and its terrifying consequences" (Federal Emergency Management Agency, 2009).

Disasters, whether caused by acts of nature or people, have been a consistent part of human history. In response to disasters and the need for emergency services, individuals, families, neighborhoods, communities, cities, states, regions, and countries have developed an organized set of responses to provide assistance and support.

One of the most well-known organizations that serves individuals and communities with disaster prevention and disaster recovery throughout the world is the Red Cross. The idea for this organization was based on the actions of a Swiss man, Henry Dunant, who, in 1859 encountered 40,000 men on a battlefield in Solferino, Italy. He mobilized locals to tend to the wounded. After this effort, Dunant encouraged the development of national organizations to provide help for those injured in war. The International Red Cross was established in 1863 to provide nonpartisan aid to wounded soldiers. The American Red Cross, founded by Clara Barton in 1881 to serve the United States in peace and war, expanded the original wartime focus to include armed forces emergency services such as communication, financial support, counseling, personnel, biomedical services, blood, tissue, plasma, and testing. The Red Cross also provides services for communities to meet needs such as food and nutrition, housing for the homeless, transportation, care for seniors, hospitals/nursing homes, youth services, and disaster services. Health and safety services such as swimming and water safety instruction, HIV/AIDS education, and youth programs support its preventive efforts (American Red Cross, 2009).

Another major emergency relief agency in the United States is the Federal Emergency Management Agency (FEMA). Founded in 1979, it became part of the Department of Homeland Security in 2003. FEMA offers education programs for adults and children on disaster preparedness. These programs help individuals develop their own family survival kits and disaster plans. In response to community disasters, FEMA offers public assistance programs to help state and local governments respond to emergencies and then recover from them. Since 1980, 52 weather-related disasters have each caused more than $1 billion in damages in the United States. Representing a variety of natural disasters, these events encompass tropical storms, hail and tornadoes, drought/heat waves, western fire seasons, hurricanes, flooding, ice storms, blizzards, and firestorms. Once an area is declared a disaster site by FEMA, a disaster recovery center (DRC) is established where individuals can meet with government officials and volunteers to express their needs and receive services (Federal Emergency Management Agency, 2009).

Frequent questions that individuals ask during a disaster indicate the pressures, stresses, and issues they face. According to FEMA, the requests focus on three sets of questions: "How can I ...?," "Where can I ...?," "What if ...?". For example, individuals want to know how they can apply for disaster assistance, get in touch with their family, or afford to rebuild. They also request information about where they can get food and water, find a place to stay, or receive crisis counseling.

"What if I lost my job?," "What if I don't have any insurance?," or "What if I need legal help?" are also common questions asked of FEMA workers (Federal Emergency Management Agency, 2009).

One particularly important need in the aftermath of a disaster is mental health support and recovery. Because loss is an inherent component during and after a disaster, many individuals and families may need short-term crisis counseling or longer-term support. In the aftermath of the September 11th terrorist

---

BOX 4.1   EVACUATION: MORE COMMON THAN YOU REALIZE

Evacuations are more common than many people realize. Hundreds of times each year, transportation and industrial accidents release harmful substances, forcing thousands of people to leave their homes.

Fires and flood cause evacuations even more frequently. Almost every year, people along the Gulf and Atlantic coasts evacuate in the face of approaching hurricanes.

Evacuation Guidelines

Always:

Keep a full tank of gas in your car if an evacuation seems likely. Gas stations may be closed during emergencies and unable to pump gas during power outages. Plan to take one car per family to reduce congestion and delay.

If time permits:
Gather your disaster supplies kit.

Make transportation arrangements with friends or your local government if you do not own a car.

Wear sturdy shoes and clothing that provides some protection, such as long pants, long-sleeved shirts, and a cap.

Listen to a battery-powered radio and follow local evacuation instructions.

Secure your home:
Close and lock doors and windows.
Unplug electrical equipment, such as radios and televisions, and small appliances, such as toasters and microwaves. Leave freezers and refrigerators plugged in unless there is a risk of flooding.

Gather your family and go if you are instructed to evacuate immediately.

Let others know where you are going.

Leave early enough to avoid being trapped by severe weather.

Follow recommended evacuation routes. Do not take shortcuts; they may be blocked.

Be alert for washed-out roads and bridges. Do not drive into flooded areas.

Stay away from downed power lines.

Other disaster preparedness information is available at https://www2.fema.gov/plan/index.shtm. For example, you will find information about a family communications plan, insurance and vital records, utilities shut off, and information for pet owners.

attacks on the World Trade Center and the Pentagon, the Substance Abuse and Mental Health Service Administration (SAMHSA) staff developed material to support emotional care and stress management. Recognizing the complexities of providing services, SAMHSA developed material for children, adolescents, parents, adults, and helping professionals. All materials included the signs or symptoms of stress in reaction to terrorist events and suggested methods of coping and providing help (Substance Abuse and Mental Health Service Administration, 2009).

CASE STUDY: MEET THE MCNEARY FAMILY

LIST OF CHARACTERS

Bill McNeary—runs a small paper supply and printing business in the southeastern United States coastal area

Nancy McNeary—co-owner of paper supply and printing business and wife of Bill

Rae McNeary—daughter of Bill and Nancy and fifth grader at the local middle school

Scott McNeary—son of Bill and Nancy and senior at the local high school

Caesar—the McNeary family dog

Hurricane Helena—Category 5 hurricane that struck the southeastern U.S. coast

THE CASE The following case study documents an actual coastal community in the southeastern United States after being hit by a hurricane. As you read this case, you will learn about the devastation that hurricanes can cause to individuals and communities. The effects of hurricanes can be both physical and emotional, and both immediate and long term.

Rae McNeary and her family moved to the coast two summers ago. Rae's father, Bill, had grown up in a beachfront house, and when his father had died, the house and his business were left to Bill. Rae had visited every summer that she could remember. She loved the salt air, the echoing crash of the waves, and the long row of houses along the sand. When her parents decided to move there permanently, she grew more and more excited. However, for Bill and his wife Nancy, the decision wasn't an easy one. Financially, it was a risk. Bill held a steady job as manager of a sawmill and Nancy was a substitute teacher. Each had dreams of running their own business one day. The paper supply/printing shop owned by Bill's father in town was a step in that direction. His father had had the place for nearly 15 years, since an early "official" retirement, which coincided with his wife's illness and death. Although not a booming business, it had done well enough to fully support the elder Mr. McNeary. Bill and Nancy made moving plans and within two years after moving had introduced new paper items to the business such as wrapping paper and greeting cards.

Rae was getting excited about starting the fifth grade. Her brother Scott was excited too, because he had finally saved enough money from summer jobs and paper routes to buy a car. It was a dumpy, old car to Rae, but nevertheless, now

Scott could drive to high school during his senior year. When Scott wasn't in school or working, he was surfing. His father continually laughed at even the thought of surfing in the southeastern coastal waters, not to mention what it actually looked like. Whenever a storm approached, Scott and his surfing buddies would hit the beach as the waves rolled in, each one darker and larger than the one before. Since they had been on the island, none of the storms had posed any threat to their area. But Bill made sure that his family was well-prepared for a hurricane. He also intrigued the children with his stories about hurricanes that had struck the southeastern coast when he was a boy.

DAY 1: MONDAY *The eighth hurricane of this season was brought to the McNearys' attention on Monday. The news that Hurricane Helena had plowed through the Virgin Islands had reached local papers and television. Leaving 14 people dead and thousands homeless, its 140 mph winds ripped apart the lush, tropical paradise found in the Caribbean. At this point, Bill began to plot its coordinates (longitude and latitude) so that he could personally keep up with where it was headed. He and Nancy reviewed the hurricane watch checklist.*

Bill knew enough about hurricanes to take them seriously. Each year the U.S. hurricane season lasts from June 1st to November 30th. Hurricanes are usually born in the warm, late-summer Atlantic Ocean waters. The steamy atmosphere that develops when ocean water quickly evaporates and combines with strong winds is the perfect environment for hurricanes to begin. They generally start as a group of thunderstorms and gradually build strength. These storms are classified by wind strength and are graded accordingly.

Hurricane Classifications

Tropical Depression	winds up to 38 mph
Tropical Storm	39 to 73 mph
Category 1	74 to 95 mph
Category 2	96 to 110 mph
Category 3	111 to 130 mph
Category 4	131 to 155 mph
Category 5	155 mph and up

For Scott and Rae, hurricane talk on the island was old business. In school, they studied how the winds around a hurricane spin in a counterclockwise direction. In the very center, as it spins, heat is pulled up from the Earth creating a "hole" in the middle. This exact center is known as the "eye." Cool air is able to descend into the eye, creating calm weather. The wind on both sides of the eye, called the "eye wall," is where the greatest intensity of the hurricane lies.

Although Scott and Rae knew the entire area covered by the hurricane could be several hundred miles wide, it was hard to imagine a storm so large. The high winds sound dangerous, and they are, but the greatest risk for damage and injury comes from the storm surge. As the winds are pulled and spiral upwards, seawater is pulled up, too. By the time the hurricane hits land, it can create a wall of water more than 10 feet above normal. This storm surge causes 90 percent of the deaths in a hurricane.

DAY 2 AND DAY 3: TUESDAY AND WEDNESDAY *On the following day, Tuesday, news came that Hurricane Helena had whipped across Puerto Rico and left more than 50,000 homeless. Although it was too early for any official information about where or when the hurricane might strike the United States, Bill and Nancy sat down that evening to make a list of what they needed to do to be prepared. They were not too concerned, but the island was a barrier island, making it more susceptible to damage than inland areas. Wednesday morning, as news came that Hurricane Helena had battered the Bahamas, Bill left Nancy at the shop and went to find duct tape, masking tape, extra flashlights, batteries, candles, matches, lamp oil, and fuel for their camping stove. Even though there was only a hurricane watch in effect, not a warning, Bill began getting things ready at home. Tape was applied across the windows to prevent shattering. He stored their lawn furniture, grill, bicycles, and a few other knickknacks in the utility room. He filled empty plastic jugs with water. Bill also visited the bank for some "just in case" money, the grocery store, and the gas station. There were lines everywhere in town at the gas station, bank, grocery store, and hardware store.*

When Scott and Rae came home from school, Bill sent Scott to fill his car with gas and then to check on his mother at the shop. Scott's mind was only on one thing as he raced into town: surfing! To him, all of the commotion was kind of exciting, definitely out of the ordinary. He quickly ran the errands, got his surfboard, and took off to find his friends and hit the waves. Rae spent her afternoon tagging along with her father. She helped him move a few valuables into their attic so they would be safe. She also tried playing with Caesar, the family's Labrador retriever, but Caesar wasn't in a playing mood. He, too, sensed the unusual commotion. Everything seemed to be about waiting for the hurricane to approach.

Late that afternoon, Bill took old plywood that he had at home and headed to their shop. Nancy anxiously awaited him, as she had been watching nearby shop owners take precautionary measures. He taped and covered their glass-front store as best as he could. Nancy busied herself inside, trying to store what she could of the various paper products. When they had done all that they could, they headed home for the evening. That night they learned from television the aftermath of Hurricane Helena in the Virgin Islands, where National Guardsmen were patrolling the streets because of looting. Weather reports said that Hurricane Helena would most likely hit anywhere within a 250-mile span on the southeastern coast. The area included the McNearys' coastal town.

Although no official warning had been posted, Rae and Scott's schools closed Wednesday. Scott was thrilled, because it meant an entire day on the beach. Rae was thrilled too, but she was also more than a little scared. She had never seen the ocean as rough as it was, nor had her parents ever been as nervous either. Her father reassured her before she climbed into bed that everything would be okay. The waiting continued for the hurricane.

DAY 4: THURSDAY *Rae awoke with a start Thursday morning to her mother calling her name. The governor had ordered an evacuation of the barrier islands and coastal communities. A deputy from the County Sheriff's Department had already been by to advise the residents on their island to leave by noon. Bill and Nancy had previously decided to stay in the area. Everything they had was in their shop or their home, and to leave both was too much for them to contemplate. They*

| BOX 4.2 | HURRICANE CHECKLIST: DURING THE HURRICANE |

If a hurricane is likely in your area, you should:

- Listen to the radio or TV for information.
- Secure your home, close storm shutters, and secure outdoor objects or bring them indoors.
- Turn off utilities if instructed to do so. Otherwise, turn the refrigerator thermostat to its coldest setting and keep its doors closed.
- Turn off propane tanks. Avoid using the phone, except for serious emergencies.
- Moor your boat if time permits.
- Ensure a supply of water for sanitary purposes such as cleaning and flushing toilets. Fill the bathtub and other large containers with water.

You should evacuate under the following conditions:

- If you are directed by local authorities to do so. Be sure to follow their instructions.
- If you live in a mobile home or temporary structure—such shelters are particularly hazardous during hurricanes no matter how well fastened to the ground.

- If you live in a high-rise building—hurricane winds are stronger at higher elevations.
- If you live on the coast, on a floodplain, near a river, or on an inland waterway.
- If you feel you are in danger.

If you are unable to evacuate, go to your safe room. If you do not have one, follow these guidelines:

- Stay indoors during the hurricane and away from windows and glass doors.
- Close all interior doors—secure and brace external doors.
- Keep curtains and blinds closed. Do not be fooled if there is a lull; it could be the eye of the storm—winds will pick up again.
- Take refuge in a small interior room, closet, or hallway on the lowest level.
- Lie on the floor under a table or another sturdy object.

From: Federal Emergency Management Agency. (2007). Hurricane. http://www.fema.gov/hazard/hurricane/index.shtm.

---

called Nancy's sister in Michigan to let her know of their plans to go to one of the designated shelters. Scott was upset at first about not getting to surf the huge waves, but he was beginning to feel uneasy about the whole situation. He and Rae rechecked stored items and picked out a few personal valuables to put in the attic. They packed items for their overnight stay at the shelter, and Bill rounded up insurance and bank papers along with birth certificates.

Nancy cleaned their bathtubs and filled them with water in case it was needed upon their return after Hurricane Helena. Bill took down the television antenna and put it in the garage along with Scott's car, lowered the garage door, and braced it. Finally, they covered their refrigerator and freezer with blankets to delay thawing. Nancy was worried about all their food, but if they were back by tomorrow, then everything should be all right. The last item on their list of things to take care of before they left was to turn off the utilities: electricity, gas, and water. Rae had spent the last hour calling Caesar in order to say goodbye. The shelters didn't allow pets, and all the kennels they had called were full. When Caesar didn't show up, Bill told Rae that Caesar was a smart dog and could take care of himself. They left lots of food and water for him, just in case. Rae thought of Caesar all alone, and big tears rolled down her face. She watched their house disappear from view as they drove away.

Area schools had been designated as shelters. The McNearys decided to go into town and do a few last minute things to their shop. The shop bore the name of Island Paper and Print and was located near the historic district on Front Street. Besides being a tourist area, locals knew many of the established businesses and patronized them. The street faced the river, making it especially vulnerable to water damage, but everyone had prepared the best they could. When the McNearys arrived at the high school, almost 300 people had signed in. It had opened at 10:00 A.M. that morning, and people had trickled in all day. Armed with blankets, pillows, a cooler, and some things to keep themselves occupied, they found a spot where they could "set up camp" for the evening. Along with hundreds of other people, the McNeary family would face Hurricane Helena.

The night of the hurricane was a nightmare. The wind roared for hours, trees snapped and crashed, transformers exploded, and rain blew sideways in sheets; rescue vehicles became stranded, roofs blew off shelters, and power lines whipped in the wind. The school shuddered and vibrated under the strain. An eerie quiet fell with the early morning. Thinking the nightmare was over, Rae saw people drift outside, not knowing that the hurricane had really just begun.

THE AFTERMATH *At the high school, reports began to pour in from all over the island. Overall, the town had survived quite well. Most of the damage came from fallen trees on power lines and broken windows. The town's famous historic district was the hardest hit. Heavy roof damage to several homes and many downed trees prompted the police to seal off the district. Residents, business owners, and emergency personnel were the only ones allowed access. Police patrolled the streets to prevent looting. Historic Front Street, which faced the river, received a lot of damage when the river rose over eight feet above normal.*

Since residents had no power, a dusk-to-dawn curfew was in effect until 24 hours after electricity was restored to the whole city—an estimated three to five days. City officials did make plans to hook up an emergency power plant to the city system so that the hospital, along with police, fire, and some commercial food and supply stores, could receive electricity.

THE MCNEARY FAMILY'S PERSPECTIVE *For Bill and Nancy McNeary and their two children, the hurricane was devastating in so many ways. When they were finally allowed back on the island, they found that their home was severely damaged. In fact, it was uninhabitable. Only those with proof of ownership were permitted on the island and then, only during daylight hours. Since the McNearys had been away for four days, the refrigerated food had spoiled and their home suffered extensive water damage—none of their furniture or belongings were salvageable. Nancy cried as she climbed over debris. Rae called and called Caesar to no avail, and she began to sob, fearing the worst. To Scott, it still seemed a great adventure as he wondered when he could get back to surfing. Bill, overcome with the destruction of the island, stared dejectedly at the ocean. They were not alone in their despair. Nothing on the island was habitable and their friends and neighbors shared the grief over the loss of their homes.*

Unfortunately, the shop had fared no better. Located on Front Street in the town's historic district where the river had flooded, the paper supply and printing shop had extensive water damage, ruining the majority of their paper products and printing machinery. Bill knew at a glance the shop was gone. He didn't believe their insurance was sufficient to cover these losses.

At this point, they could only think about their immediate consequences. The McNearys had to find a temporary place to live until they could decide what to do. They only had food and the belongings they had taken with them to the shelter. Physically, their basic needs were met, but they were overwhelmed by so many other concerns. Financial worries began to weigh on them as they dealt with their other losses.

ONE MONTH LATER *With help from the American Red Cross, FEMA, and local agencies, the McNearys were living in a mobile home until they could decide what to do about their house. Although conditions were crowded, Nancy felt they were all lucky to have what they had and to be alive. Admittedly, her relationship with Bill was strained. His depression at the loss of both home and business coupled with the frustrations of the seemingly endless forms for both FEMA and insurance made each evening meal tense. They didn't seem to talk anymore. Nancy needed to share with him her concerns about Scott and Rae, and she needed to talk with him about what was happening to them as a couple. She knew he was stressed but so was she. Adding to the strain was their son Scott's hyperactivity. While Bill was increasingly quiet and withdrawn, Scott was literally bouncing his basketball off the wall, playing loud music, and being argumentative. He couldn't seem to settle down. Nancy's frustration and helplessness about what was happening to her family caused her to overlook Rae, who seemed almost invisible. She was quiet and passive, volunteering little information about school, friends, her feelings, or the hurricane. She caused no trouble and did what she was asked.*

Nancy wondered if she and Bill were handling the aftermath of the hurricane correctly, especially where the children were concerned. They had taken them to the island the first time, but the widespread destruction was so upsetting that they didn't take them back. Their schools were closed due to hurricane damage and both Scott and Rae were temporarily in new schools with new classmates. Nancy knew the teachers and counselors were making efforts to help the students deal with the effects of the hurricane through art, class discussions, sharing, and guidance groups. She thought both Scott and Rae were finding this helpful. But how did she know? And Bill did not talk to Scott and Rae much anymore. For a week he had been working for the local power company on their emergency crew team. He left home at 6:00 A.M. and returned at 8:00 P.M. exhausted from his long day. He ate a late supper and excused himself to get ready for bed.

Nancy was finding it increasingly difficult to sleep at night and even harder to control her anger at Bill for not helping with the family. She knew he was doing his best, but she and the kids needed his emotional support. She felt as if everything was falling apart around her and she couldn't stop it from happening. After one particularly ugly exchange with Bill one morning, she got everyone off to school and work and sat down for a good cry. Although she felt somewhat better, she immediately made an appointment with her doctor. Knowing that she had taken at least one step toward taking action made her feel a bit more positive.

Dr. Landon listened carefully as Nancy described how she felt and what was going on at home. He talked with her about the hurricane, the devastation, and her physical and emotional reactions. He suggested she take an antidepressant for a limited time and referred her to a mental health center for counseling. The staff of the mental health center, realizing that so many people needed help dealing with the effects of the hurricane, had formed several support groups for children, youth, young women, couples, and retirees. Dr. Landon felt that Nancy would benefit from talking with other wives and mothers about their situations. Many of the reactions Nancy shared with him were similar to those who had survived the hurricane. He suggested that at some point Bill might consider joining her in the couples' group. Based on his visit with Nancy, he was a bit concerned about the other family members and suggested she call him in one week to report how they were doing.

By the time Nancy arrived home, she was feeling much better. Then she noticed a message on the answering machine. It was the school counselor asking Nancy to call her back as soon as possible. Nancy discovered that Rae had arrived at school that morning, but no one had seen her after recess. How in the world could this happen? How could the school lose a child? In a panic, Nancy called Bill and he agreed to meet her at the school. When they arrived, they met with the principal, the school counselor, and a security officer who was in touch with the police department. The school had already provided the police with a description of Rae and an alert was broadcast.

Approximately 45 minutes later, a police officer arrived with Rae. The officer had seen her at the bus stop, and because she was not in school, stopped to see if everything was all right. Rae informed her she was taking the bus to the island to look for Caesar, her dog. She was worried and afraid that something had happened to him. When they arrived at the school, Rae and her parents talked with the school counselor. Nancy and Bill were so relieved; they hugged and kissed Rae repeatedly. The school counselor sensed that communication was not working among the three of them so she encouraged them to come into her office to talk about their problems. The school counselor was able to get Rae to tell her parents how she felt, particularly her worries and fears about Caesar.

The counselor also talked with the McNearys about some of the stresses families were experiencing after the hurricane—added bills, a temporary home, longer work hours, and the loss of cherished belongings. For Scott and Rae, the stresses included a new school, new friends, the crowded mobile home, and the loss of Caesar, favorite belongings, and the familiar. She also explained that even though the teachers and other school staff encouraged students to talk about their experiences and their feelings, often problems don't show up for several months. Rae had attempted to do something about her problems. More than that, she had alerted both her parents and school staff that she needed their help.

CASE QUESTIONS

1. List *all* of the services provided before, during, and after Hurricane Helena.

_____

_____

_____

_____

_____

_____

_____

_____

2. Using the list prepared in Question 1, identify each service as medical, public
    health, or human service model. Describe the characteristics of each service
    that relate to the model you choose.

_____

_____

_____

_____

_____

_____

_____

3. List the problems the McNearys face after the hurricane.

_____

_____

_____

_____

_____

_____

4. Describe in detail the emotional impact of a natural disaster upon the
    McNearys.

_____

_____

_____

_____

_____

_____

_____

_____

5. What problems do you think will remain for the McNearys one year after the hurricane?

_____

_____

_____

_____

_____

_____

_____

_____

6. For the problems you listed in Question 5, describe which models of service delivery will be most effective in supporting this family. Be specific about the services they will need.

_____

_____

_____

_____

_____

_____

_____

_____

EXERCISE: YOU AS THE HUMAN SERVICE PROFESSIONAL

Now that you have an understanding of the three models of service delivery and are familiar with the devastation of a natural disaster like a hurricane and the difficulties that result, answer the following questions:

1. What is your reaction to this case?

_____

_____

_____

_____

_____

_____

_____

_____

2. What do you think are the challenges working with clients who need
    emergency services?

_____

_____

_____

_____

_____

_____

_____

3. How would you use the human service model to deliver emergency
    services?

_____

_____

_____

_____

_____

_____

_____

4. What qualities or characteristics do you have that would help you work
    effectively in disaster relief?

_____

_____

_____

_____

_____

_____

_____

_____

5. What would be most difficult for you?

_____

_____

_____

_____

_____

_____

_____

ANOTHER PERSPECTIVE: HOLLY STULTS AND PATRICK FITZSIMMONS

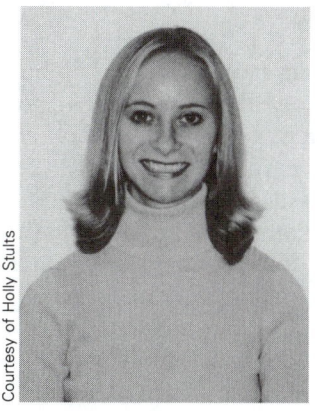

Courtesy of Holly Stults

This perspective has two authors. Holly Stults, a Human Service graduate, completed her field experience at the American Red Cross. Her job responsibilities included working with disaster services, intake and case management, maintaining a database of client information, performing screening and assessment of military-related cases, and verification and reporting of messages for armed forces emergency services. She attends graduate school in health administration. Patrick Fitzsimmons, her supervisor, has been the Direct Services Administrator for the American Red Cross for 18 years. His responsibilities include managing disaster relief and service to military families and overseeing and conducting health and safety training programs. Holly and Patrick describe the work of Carol Burcham, who directs the American Red Cross chapter involved in this case.

The case study tells the story of the McNeary family during Hurricane Helena. The following is a behind-the-scenes account of disaster relief as experienced by an employee of the American Red Cross.

Carol Burcham is the director of the local chapter of the American Red Cross whose service area includes the island affected by Hurricane Helena. Carol has had three days to prepare for the hurricane. The national headquarters of the Red

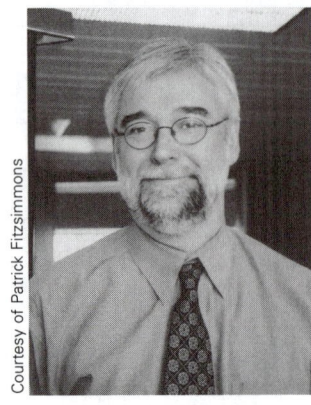

Courtesy of Patrick Fitzsimmons

Cross has set up a staging area in Atlanta where several emergency response vehicles (ERVs) and plenty of staff are waiting until after the storm passes. They will descend on the area immediately after the storm and set up a relief operation. Until then, Carol is dependent upon local resources for the most part.

Since she did have a few days to prepare, Carol had extra cots, clean-up kits, and comfort kits shipped to the chapter in advance so she was sure to have enough once disaster struck. Clean-up kits contain a mop, bucket, broom, bleach, and other supplies to help victims clean up their home after a disaster. Comfort kits include personal toiletry items such as soap, toothpaste, deodorant, shampoo, a razor, and shaving cream.

Carol contacted several other local agencies to talk about how they would coordinate their efforts when needed. She made arrangements in advance to open eight shelters in the county for evacuees. Since she knew she would not have enough round-the-clock staff to manage these shelters, she implemented an agreement she had previously made with the local Council of Churches for extra staff. These people had already been trained in shelter operations. With the help of these extra volunteers, Red Cross staff and volunteers, and the help of clients in the shelters, the shelters would run smoothly. Carol expected to have approximately 200 people in each shelter. The shelters would be set up inside local schools. Therefore, their foodstuffs could be used for the shelters, and the Red Cross would then reimburse the school system for what was used.

DAY OF THE HURRICANE

On the day of the approaching hurricane, families begin coming into the shelters. Each family must register, and trained volunteers are on hand to move the process along smoothly. Because there are so few volunteers at each shelter, clients who wish to help are quickly trained in the intake process.

The importance of Carol's pre-disaster networking soon becomes apparent. Many families have brought their pets along. Some families have cats or dogs; this could easily turn into a disaster in itself. Luckily, the local Humane Society has donated food and kennels to keep all the animals separated.

Once things begin to settle down, Carol and her staff begin assigning work to volunteers as well as shelter clients. Based on their abilities, people are assigned to cooking, cleaning, first aid, management, and security duties. Red Cross mental health workers circulate among the clients providing some support, but mainly they just provide a sympathetic ear. People here are afraid, and many of them just need to express their fears to someone.

DAY AFTER THE STORM

Once the storm passes, American Red Cross volunteers trained in damage assessment hit the streets. The responsibilities of the damage assessment team are manifold. These volunteers help physically plan the operation by providing information about safe routes and open roads that can be used by volunteers providing mass care. They also monitor weather forecasts so as to predict areas that could be susceptible to flooding. The work of the damage assessment volunteers will help Carol with several activities. The information the damage assessment volunteers provide will help in determining the most urgent needs and in setting priorities for providing assistance. The assessment will help determine staffing and supply needs, and it will help estimate relief costs, which will in turn lead to a basis for fund-raising decisions. Of course, it is also the job of the damage assessment volunteers to verify the damage suffered by those who request assistance from the Red Cross.

Shelter workers begin passing out the clean-up kits that they had stockpiled. More trained Red Cross volunteers head out in ERVs to begin mobile feeding operations in the affected areas. Each ERV has a particular route, and they stop for anyone that they see along the way. People who are working on cleaning up their homes, the National Guard, and other emergency workers can get meals or snacks without leaving their posts. Besides providing food, the volunteers in the ERVs also hand out clean-up kits. They are trained to provide clients with information about where to go for assistance, and they relay information to their supervisors about additional services or supplies needed.

Fixed feeding sites remain open at the shelters, and volunteers organize games and activities for the children whose parents have gone to assess damage and start on clean-up. Carol assesses her needs for the relief operation and communicates with the staging area in Atlanta. Incoming staff is oriented at a headquarters facility and volunteers begin fund-raising efforts.

Two or More Days after the Storm

Now the real casework begins. Carol sets up a service center at a local church to provide family services to hurricane victims. The immediate needs that must be met are for clothing and shelter; many families' clothing has been ruined even if their homes have not. Family service caseworkers take their information and begin case files on these affected families. The caseworkers issue vouchers for clothing, made out to local stores that already have an agreement with the Red Cross. While the Red Cross cannot assist in the search for those who will need to find new homes, they can assist with the first month's rent, provided the family can continue to pay the rent after the first month. Once these families do find new homes, the Red Cross can issue more vouchers to cover bedding, linens, dinette sets, and kitchenware. On some occasions, the Red Cross may even help with the purchase of a refrigerator or stove.

Fixed feeding sites remain open, and mobile feeding operations continue throughout the community. Once power has been restored, those whose houses have been declared safe and clear are encouraged to move out of the shelter and return to their homes. Volunteers continue their fund-raising efforts.

As more people are allowed back into their homes, shelters are shut down and residents are consolidated. Hotlines are set up and staffed around the clock to provide answers to disaster victims' questions about recovery and resources. The volunteers who have come from other cities, counties, and states begin to go home as the caseload becomes progressively smaller.

Now that most everyone's immediate needs have been attended to, some of the most important Red Cross volunteers are those trained in accounting. These volunteers handle all of the vouchers, or dispersing orders, as they come in from the merchants, and process them for payment. These volunteers keep track of all the funds that are spent on the disaster relief operation. Not only do they track the funds, but they also maintain the records of services provided, quantities served, and supplies used. The chapter will send a daily report to the national headquarters until all of the cases have been closed.

From providing shelters to tallying up bills, the few weeks since the disaster felt more like months. Carol found it hard to believe that a simple force of nature could take so much from people in so many different ways. Not only did it take away many families' homes and possessions, but it also took an enormous amount of money to assist in recovery. It took hundreds of hours of work on the part of everyone involved. More than anything, it took courage, generosity, and cooperation from both victims and volunteers. These things made recovery truly possible.

EXERCISE: THE LAST WORD

You have the opportunity to have the last word on the terms introduced and the case study presented. Based on what you have learned in this chapter, answer the following questions.

1. When you think about what you have read about the models of service delivery, what stands out for you?

_____

_____

_____

_____

_____

_____

_____

2. How did the chapter change your ideas and understanding about how services are delivered?

_____

_____

_____

_____

_____

_____

_____

_____

3. How will you use the information in this chapter in your own life and work?

_____

_____

_____

_____

_____

_____

_____

_____

4. What questions remain unanswered for you?

_____

_____

_____

_____

_____

_____

_____

_____

FOR FURTHER STUDY

BOOKS

Brennan, V. M. (2009). *Natural disasters and public health: Hurricanes Katrina, Rita, and Wilma*. Baltimore, MD: The Johns Hopkins Press. Reports from the field by disaster relief professionals and research articles by scholars present lessons learned from these hurricanes and offer guidance for the future.

Clements, B. (2009). *Disasters and public health: Planning and response*. Oxford, UK: Butterworth-Heinemann. Based upon years of experience as an expert in public health and disaster medical assistance, the author has researched and compiled information about planning and response to disasters from wildfires to multi-drug resistant strains of bacteria.

Hemingway, L. (2002). *A world turned over: A killer tornado and the lives it changed forever*. Upper Saddle River, NJ: Simon & Schuster. The grand-daughter of Ernest Hemingway tells in her own words and those of the survivors the story of the devastating tornado that struck Candlestick Shopping Center in South Jackson, Mississippi, on March 3, 1966. The author describes how a familiar setting is turned into a morass of concrete, glass, metal, cars, and broken bodies.

Junger, Sebastian (1999). *The perfect storm: A true story of men against the sea*. New York: Perennial. A rare combination of factors created a "perfect storm" that hit North America's eastern seaboard in October 1991. This book details the meteorological conditions and the impact the storm had on many of the people caught in it.

Maclean, John N. (1999). *Fire on the mountain: The true story of the South Canyon Fire*. New York: William Morrow. The catastrophic South Canyon fire of 1994 burned for 12 days and cost approximately $4.5 million and the lives of 14 firefighters.

Ramroth, W. (2007). *Planning for disaster: How natural and manmade disasters shape the built environment*. New York: Kaplan Business. This book references a myriad of disasters to describe how they impact the building design of projects such as bridges, tunnels, and levees. The Oklahoma City bombing (1995), the 9/11 terrorist attack (2001), as well as earlier events such as the burning of Rome (AD 64) and the Great Chicago Fire of 1871 are examples.

Reisner, Marc (2003). *A dangerous place: California's unsettling fate*. New York: Pantheon. The author offers an assessment of the future of California, which rests on grave geological instability. He combines a history of Los Angeles's and San Francisco's growth with a scenario of what the San Francisco Bay area will be like after the "big one."

Schaefer, M. (2007). *Lost in Katrina*. Greta, La.: Pelican Publishing Co. The residents of St. Bernard's parish were among the hardest hit by Hurricane Katrina. Their own words provide personal stories about the first seven days of the disaster.

Steinberg, T. (2006). *Acts of god: The unnatural history of natural disaster in America*. New York: Oxford University Press USA. The author examines how natural disasters arrive from nature, but it is the social and cultural context of America that turns them into disasters.

Yuvell, N., Galea, S., & Norris, F. H. (2009). *Mental health and disasters*. New York: Cambridge University Press. Since September 11th, the mental health component of disaster response has received a great deal of attention. This book serves as a reference on disasters and mental health.

MOVIES

9/11 (2002). Directors: Gédéon Naudet, and James Hanlon. Documentary of the firefighters who battled the fires at Ground Zero when the planes crashed into the World Trade Center.

NOVA—Hurricane Katrina: The Storm that Drowned a City. (2006). Director: Nova. Actors: Stacy Keach, Peter Thomas (VI), and Don Wescott, This hour-by-hour reconstruction of Hurricane Katrina exposes the failures in preparation and engineering that led to the worst disaster in American history.

The River (1984). Director: Mark Rydell. Starring: Mel Gibson, Sissy Spacek. Tom Garvey (Mel Gibson) and his wife Mae (Sissy Spacek) own a small farm in east Tennessee that has been in the family for generations. The family faces several hardships in this movie including severe storms and threatened repossession by the bank.

WEB SITES

Explore the Web to learn more about the following:

American Red Cross
Salvation Army
Federal Emergency Management Agency (FEMA)
Disaster Relief Emergency Assistance Act

disaster
hurricane(s)
public health
social services

REFERENCES

American Red Cross. (2009) *Home*. Retrieved from the http://www.redcross.org/.

Federal Emergency Management Agency. (2009). *About FEMA*. Retrieved from http://www.fema.gov.

Substance Abuse and Mental Health Service Administration. (2009). *About SAMHSA*. Retrieved from http://www.samhsa.gov/.

THE CLIENT

The focus of Chapter 5 is the client, one of the participants in the helping process and the recipient of human services. Within the human service context, clients are individuals, families, communities, or larger geographic areas. They become clients in the human service delivery system because they have needs they are unable to meet, problems they cannot resolve, or both. Who are they? How do they become clients? What kinds of needs or problems do they experience? You will explore questions like these as you read this chapter.

This chapter begins by asking you to think about what it means to live near or below the poverty line. You will use key concepts from Chapter 5 of your textbook *Introduction to Human Services, 7th ed.* Next, you will describe a time when you faced problems, issues, and challenges. Then, we define several key ideas to help you understand clients and their problems and explore how people get help from human service agencies, organizations, and professionals. In order to apply this knowledge, you will read about teenage gangs to prepare for a case study on Alphonse, an inner-city gang member. Understanding the key ideas and applying them to Alphonse's case will increase your knowledge of human service clients. Questions for you to think about follow the case study. A human service professional then reviews Alphonse's case. Finally, resources you can use for future study conclude the chapter.

INTRODUCTION

The following exercise will assist you in understanding what it means to live at the poverty line by exploring the limited choices that result from poverty. This activity has several steps, and it will be helpful to work with other students to form a family group (4–7 members). As a group, complete the following assignments.

1. Find the current poverty guideline by checking The website Housing Works, 2009 to 2010 Federal Poverty Guidelines. Describe the process by which the guidelines were originally established.
2. According to the formula, it is recommended that one-third of income is used for food. As an example, for a family of six, assume the poverty line is

approximately \$29,530. Thus, \$9,843 annually is available for food purchase. To determine how much money is available for one dinner, divide by the number of days during the year and then, (somewhat arbitrarily) decide that half of a day's allotment ought to go for dinner.

3. Divide your family group into two equal groups, each with half of the allotment to spend in order to buy dinner for their half of the group. One half of your group will go to a local convenience store within walking distance to purchase food for dinner. The other half of your group will drive to any supermarket of their choice.

4. Both groups return with a list of their purchases and the total cost. Predicted outcomes are that the group that goes to the convenience store discovers that they have few choices (i.e., meatless spaghetti sauce in a jar and spaghetti, milk, and bread). Those who shop at the supermarket have more choices at less cost (McKinney, 2002, pp. 138–9).

EXERCISE: WHAT ABOUT YOU?

Think about your past and identify a time in your life when you experienced a series of difficulties, problems, and challenges. They can be large or small, short term or long term. Describe the situation.

_____

_____

_____

_____

_____

_____

_____

_____

KEY IDEAS

Critical to understanding human services is recognizing the complexity of client problems; sensitivity to clients' feelings about help; client attitudes, values, culture, and strengths; and the need to work with other professionals and agencies. The following key ideas will help you understand clients and their needs.

PROBLEMS

Problems are part of daily life. Everyone has problems and the potential to be a client. A problem is a situation, event, or condition that causes trouble. It may be internal, for example, an illness or a disability, or external, such as an economic downturn or a company's decision to lay off workers. Problems may also result from interpersonal situations, such as difficulties getting along with friends, family, or coworkers. People who lack the resources or skills to solve their problems often become clients. Many times an individual has more than one problem, and the problems may be so overwhelming that he or she cannot cope with any of them.

Problem and Strengths Identification

Successful helping depends upon an accurate definition of the client's problems and identifying strengths of the client and the client's situation. But both problem identification and strengths identification can be challenging. First, the helper's ability to accurately identify a problem is a contributing factor to his or her effectiveness. In human services, this effectiveness means understanding that a problem can be simple, such as a request for information, or complex, such as anger management. The client's perception of the problem must also be taken into account as should the values of the client and the client's culture. When the client and the human service professional or society do not agree that a behavior or an attitude, for example, is a problem, then the situation becomes more complicated. Identifying strengths can be equally as challenging. Clients may be so devastated they cannot see any strengths that they possess or can count on within their circumstances. They also may fear that if they identify strengths, then help will not be available to them. If clients can see how strengths have helped them succeed in the past, they may be more ready to access those strengths again.

The Whole Person

Underlying the establishment of a helping relationship and the identification of the problem is the commitment of the helper to the concept of the whole person. Not only does the helper recognize the many components that are part of the client (e.g., biological, psychological, educational, social, vocational, and spiritual), but the helper also appreciates the role of the environment in the client's situation. The complexity of who clients are and the environment in which they live, coupled with the many aspects of problems, require the helper to understand several different conceptual frameworks in order to grasp both the problem and the person.

The Developmental Approach

Several conceptual frameworks contribute to the understanding of clients and problems. The developmental framework is helpful in human services. Although a number of developmental theories exist, most agree that individuals engage in certain tasks at different points in life. Development is a process, and while individuals move through the same stages, they may experience a stage in different ways and within a different time frame. Using a developmental perspective to view problems helps human service professionals with a basic understanding of the process of growth and change that individuals normally experience.

Situational Approach

Another approach to viewing problems is situational. Situational problems occur with no predictability; an individual experiences this type of problem because he or she is at a particular place at a particular time. The individual may or may not contribute or cause situational problems. A traffic accident, a rape, a home invasion, and divorce are examples of situational problems.

BASIC HUMAN NEEDS

Thinking about basic human needs is yet another way to consider problems. Maslow's hierarchy of needs has the most fundamental physical human needs at its base. Building upon this base are safety, social needs, self-esteem, and finally, self-actualization. Basic to the model is that lower order needs must be met before addressing higher order needs. For example, a client who has not eaten in three days must have his or her hunger satisfied (a lower order need) before considering work on his or her self-esteem issues (a higher order need).

SOCIETAL CHANGE

A final conceptual framework responds to the changes occurring in the world today. In some cases, individuals experience problems not just because they have needs as human beings, but because of rapid social change that may leave them unemployed, homeless, or experiencing conflicts between old and new values. Societal change occurs rapidly—sometimes explosively—and people may find themselves in unfamiliar situations. In some cases, change can be immobilizing, particularly if an individual does not have the self-confidence, skills, or support to adjust to rapid changes.

GETTING HELP

Those who need assistance become involved in the human service system in several ways. *Voluntary clients* are those who seek services themselves or are referred by a human service professional. On the other hand, *involuntary clients* receive services which are mandated by the courts or some other official body. These clients have no choice about services and frequently challenge helpers because of their resistance. A third type of client, an *inadvertent client*, is the individual or group of individuals who receive services because they are members of a larger group targeted for services. They receive services *inadvertently* and may not even want or need the services.

BARRIERS TO HELP

The presence of barriers prevents those eligible for services from receiving them. Frequently, fear is at the root of many barriers: fear of what will happen, fear of admitting a problem exists, fear of embarrassment, and fear of human service professionals. Costs and resources are also very real problems for many clients. For example, the high cost of or lack of transportation, the lack of money, and the long travel time or distance to an agency may prevent the client from receiving help. Other less tangible costs may be psychological—loss of freedom, feelings of inadequacy, or being indebted to a human service agency or professional—and are no less real.

CLIENT EVALUATION OF SERVICES

> The emphasis on accountability today gives clients a stronger voice in the quality of services they receive. Their evaluations of services are often tied to their expectations of the human service system. Most clients come in with certain expectations of both the helper and the process. For example, they expect a helper who is unbiased, understands the client's point of view, and is competent to do whatever needs to be done. Expectations for the helping process focus on a solution to the problem.

EXERCISE: YOU AND HUMAN SERVICE CLIENTS

> The following questions focus on the issues and challenges that you described in the "What About You?" exercise at the beginning of the chapter. Review the problem(s) you described and answer the following questions.

1. List each problem you mentioned in the exercise and categorize it as developmental, situational, a basic human need, or the result of rapid social change.

_____

_____

_____

_____

_____

_____

_____

_____

2. For which difficulties did you receive help?

_____

_____

_____

_____

_____

_____

_____

_____

3. Were you a voluntary, involuntary, or inadvertent client?

_____

_____

_____

_____

_____

_____

_____

_____

4.   Did you experience any barriers to getting help?

_____

_____

_____

_____

_____

_____

_____

5.   Describe your satisfaction or dissatisfaction with the help you received.

_____

_____

_____

_____

_____

_____

_____

_____

FOCUS: INNER-CITY YOUTH GANGS

This section introduces the topic of youth gangs in the United States and provides a context for the case of Alphonse, which follows. The information will help you understand what a gang is, why young people join them, and the community efforts underway to respond to gang activity.

No one is sure exactly when or why youth gangs emerged in the United States, although their appearance may have been as early as the end of the American

Revolution. Since that time, gang proliferation has been most visible and most violent during periods of rapid immigration and population shifts. In the United States, four periods of gang growth and activity are evident: the late 1800s, the 1920s, the 1960s, and the late 1990s (Savelli, 2005).

CONCERNS

The growth of gangs in the late 1990s make youth gangs a human service concern today for several reasons. One reason is the difficulty of even assessing the scope of the problem. Confusing definitions of what constitutes a gang and denial that gangs exist in certain communities contribute to this difficulty. A second related reason is the proliferation of gangs by dividing and multiplying across the country. They also spread from schools and street level gangs to juvenile detention and correctional facilities, where gangs can also form and recruit. Violence and crime at schools and in neighborhoods and communities is also problematic. Gangs commit homicides, drive-by shootings, and other forms of violence; engage in drug trafficking and other crimes; and carry weapons. Knowing the characteristics of gangs, the attractions of gang membership, and solutions to this human service concern will help you understand the potential client groups that result from gang activity.

Youth gangs share certain characteristics. Generally, gangs develop along racial and ethnic lines and are typically male. They often display their membership through dress, colors, and specific activities and behaviors and are neighborhood or "turf" based. A gang's primary activity is the commission of criminal acts—homicide, assault with a deadly weapon, robbery, arson, and intimidation. Lieutenant Gracie Jones, a police gang specialist, offers a law enforcement definition of youth gangs:

> A gang is three or more individuals who meet all of the following. First, a gang has a name and identifiable leadership. Second, it maintains a geographical, economic, and/or criminal enterprise. Third, its members associate on a continuous or regular basis. Finally, members engage in delinquent or criminal behavior (Personal communication).

Gangs attract children and adolescents for a variety of reasons. Primarily, gangs respond to an individual's needs that are not otherwise being met—a sense of family, acceptance, status, and prestige. For many young people, the sense of alienation and powerlessness that result from the lack of traditional support structures leads to feelings of frustration and anger (Savelli, 2005). In addition, for some individuals the chance for excitement, earning money, and protection from other gangs are the motivations for joining. Gang membership provides a sense of belonging and identity as well as a sense of power and control. Its activities provide an outlet for anger. The perception of control also extends to "turf," and gangs often will use force to control both its territory and its members. While gangs recruit members, a few are born into gangs as a result of neighborhood traditions or parents' earlier (or continuing) gang participation, or both.

SOLUTIONS

Human service professionals have a number of strategies to counter gangs. Interventions in schools have been effective. These programs include preventing school-age children from initially joining gangs; special programs for parents; education about gangs, their destructiveness, and how to avoid being drawn into them; and creating a climate at school where each child feels valued and successful.

In some communities, cooperative efforts among schools, law enforcement, employers, and community agencies have resulted in collaborative approaches to gang problems. Often, such efforts combine prevention, social intervention, rehabilitation, suppression, and community mobilization.

CASE STUDY: MEET ALPHONSE

The case of Alphonse takes you into the world of a teenage gang member. You will hear about his life and his interaction with the social service system from his perspective. Because this chapter focuses on the client, it is important to understand his world and the context in which he operates. One of the most valuable ways in which helpers assist their clients is by focusing on them, understanding who they are, what strengths they have, and what help they believe they need. This focus on the client is often difficult when the client lives in a world that is measurably different from that of the helper.

LIST OF CHARACTERS

Alphonse—teenage gang member

Little Mikie—Alphonse's little brother

Zodiacs—rival gang

Bernard—member of Alphonse's gang

Ms. Parnell—Alphonse's counselor

In this case, Alphonse, a member of an inner-city gang, comes face to face with Ms. Parnell, a community counselor. Alphonse lives in a culture where the gang is his major support. Ms. Parnell attempts to work with Alphonse and this is his account of their encounter. Each gang has its own slang, symbols, clothing, and ways of identifying other members. Gang members incorporate *rap* and *hip hop* terms into their vocabularies.

The following terms and their definitions might help you better understand Alphonse's dialogue:

beasting—fighting; attacking

crew—group of friends who form a gang

dirty bottle—positive urine test

dissin'—giving someone a hard time

ho—low status

hook—the legal authorities

illing—hurting

ink—tattoo

juvie—juvenile detention home

pal—parolee

p.o.—probation officer

paper—money

rollin—making money

Please note: This case study was created from in-depth research on gangs and gang culture. **Because it is told from the client's perspective, it contains language that some readers may find offensive.**

THE CASE

APRIL 27   *My crew was right. It ain't no bullshit. I can give you plenty of nothin'. The streets are plenty crowded, but I got no fuss. Sure it look like I live with my momma, but I ain't seen her but twice this week. She always dissin' me, and I don't stay 'round much. Last night I stopped by just for nothin' and she was on my ass after I walk in the door. I stayed long enough to pick up my hat and old crew shirt, and I was gone. She'd like me better if I was rollin' like some on the streets. She not sure she like the crew, but I know she like it plenty 'specially cause I gone and don't give her no shit, and I don't ask her for no paper.*

Little Mikie, my bro', come with me tonight. He knew where the action is here in the 'hood. He had black pants on just like me, and he want to be part of the crew. Mikie only eight, but he know where the best life is. Not at home with momma bitching and hitting, better to be hit by your crew. They always be by you. Two of the crew try getting tough with Mikie, putting their hands on him. He just look at me and take it. With his gang he be beasting back, but not here. They won't hurt him bad, and it make him tough. If he's some little fag, he don't belong. He'll make it, I 'spect, cause he been getting money from school since he real young. I showed him how to get lunch money and food from the punks. Shit momma give nobody money. He don't go much anyway. Not much happen' at school 'cept seeing the crew and scoping on bitches.

Tonight we meetin' at the park. We go bust heads of the Zodiacs. They jumped on Malcolm and Jer last week at the mall. We beast on their asses for messing with our crew. We'll get anybody from that crew. We don't just go for the person who did whatever. When we cut loose with that Uzi, they know they don't mean shit to us. Their big fellas got paper and think they're shit. We might waste one or two and maybe more. The more the better. Rolando is goin' tonight. He crushes mugs and kicks ass. He'll kill any suckers in his way. A month ago he got real pissed and borrowed a Uzi and sprayed the crackhead up the street. By the time we finish, they'll know us. Mikie won't look like us—he got no jacket or tattoos or black shoes, but he cool with his black pants. He see his first beasting with the crew tonight.

MAY 12   *Tonight I got paper. Man, belonging to the crew is the only way. Bernard says he gettin' us big dough, and we hitting the big time. Without doughski you ain't shit. He rollin' now, and the bitches think he cool with his gold chains and his Benz. He says we got to be smart or the hook catch us. Some in our crew are dumb, they illing doing shit. I say we jump on them and tell them to get out. We can hit the action, if we can keep the hook out of our shit. Bernard also beasting everyone on 'caine. He say no dope fiends rollin'. I wanna be shit, so I quit. Going to school then be real fun. Show those clothes, jewelry, and things like that. Fuck goin' to school to get a job. I got a job with the crew.*

JUNE 22   *I wouldn't say things are fucked, but I'm a pal for selling 'caine. Wasn't no big sell, but the hook was there on my corner. Goin' to prison, no that don't scare me. I'm too young, and next time I won't get caught. This really ain't too bad. I'm tryin' to be cool, so I won't go to the detention home. I ain't goin' nowhere. Some say prison ain't so bad. You can get dope and anything else you want. If you don't fuck with the big man and lay low, then prison life can get you straight with the right people.*

I got this stiff-assed p.o. Time to be gettin' rid of him. He's dissing me about the crew and the dope. So far I don't give him a dirty bottle. Wants me to get a job. I tell him. I got a job. Fuck working for $4 a hour and listenin' to some motherfucker tell me what to do. I be beasting him in a minute. My p.o. sent me to see this bitch about joinin' a training program so I can get a job. So I go just to fill the time. This bitch she not as bad as some I've seen, and she not like my momma. But she sure got some stupid-ass ways of talking. I was there 30 minutes, and she tried to turn me upside down. Fuck that stuff. I told her about my crew. The crew don't need no trainin' program. She wasn't dissing me like those teachers and counselors at the school, and she didn't even say "go back to school." Good thing for her, if she'd start dissing me I'd had to jump on her.

The bitch she asked me lots of questions I answered, but I don't like nobody asking. She want to know about my momma, my pisshead father, I never knew him. I told her to leave Mikie out of it. We did laugh about school when I began beasting kids. I told her that assholes in school always dissin' me. She said she understood. She went to the same school and be living just down the street from Jer, one of my crew.

JULY 18   *The last time I saw my counselor she talked to me about problem solving. That's what she called it. Now I could tell her about being shit when you got doughski, now that's when you don't have problems. She want to know what I want. Nobody ever asked me, and I'd always say fuck them, I'll get what I want for myself. My momma never did say, "What you want?" I ain't never heard those words. So I told her I wanted doughski, cars, and bitches, and jumping on people who get in my way. All this happens with my crew. They be my family, and no problem solving take that away. And one sure-ass problem is my p.o. That is little problem, paper is big one. She call these "multiples."*

What I want? I want paper and to be shit and to be with my crew. And I got this, if my p.o. get off my ass. When this is over, I can get him later. I don't want him fucking with me.

JULY 25   *Today we meet just for a minute. I tell the bitch I ain't got much time, the crew has a meeting in 30 minutes. And I ain't shit if I'm late. She just wanted me to check in. I want her and my p.o. off my ass. I was out before she say "goodbye."*

JULY 27   *It's not me, but I like this bitch. She say today she gonna stretch my mind. I tell her not to fuck with my mind. I don't want no one messing with my mind. Some guys in prison get their minds fucked, because they get popped by the big guys. They just do what everybody says. So we made a list of every way I can get paper. She say I creative 'cause I can make up things. Then she showed me why I was so smart. My asshole list was long—and I had some fucking answers she said nobody had ever said. She had one problem, she say most are illegal.*

I had lots of fuckin' ideas on the list. But she just don't know. I'd rather stand on the corners in the rain and in the winter being tough for the crew than in them plants and silly-ass places where they treat me like ho. And my crew would beast my ass if I left them.

Making these lists, it was almost like the fun I had with that bitch teacher in school, when I was Mikie's age. We'd fuckin' yell out lots of answers. She thought we were shit, too. But that was for dumb-ass kids. My list today is shit, but the bitch laughed. She say my fuckin' p.o. would gag if he saw the list. No way to do the list and get out of the hook's way! We played "what if you could...." I couldn't get out of there without saying some dumbshit thing like "thanks." I know shit, and I know that was just a list. She really don't know. How can she talk about a better life? I know them preppy niggahs that go to college. They got no clothes and drive them ugly-ass cars. The crew calls them ho cars. My momma is proud of me. She waitin' till I bring home the big paper. I don't need no school.

At the fuckin' end of my time the bitch wanted me to pretend, "What if I had all this paper and wanted to lose it?" I tell her if I got it I ain't never losing it.

AUGUST 22   *I ain't been to see the bitch counselor in weeks, but my p.o. is on my ass. Seeing her wasn't so bad. She didn't bullshit me, and she not part of the phony-talking tight-asshole group. She got her crew, and I got mine. I guess even the mayor got his crew. He got bitches and do his dope just like us. He dissing us, but he do just like us. He jump on people and fuck the things he like. He not real. But my counselor, she real.*

She glad to see me. I felt shit seein' her, but I don't want no bullshit. She still got the list we made. You know, bullshit ways to get paper. But I lay low and listen. She still not dissin' me. Say she there for me. She should see my MAC 10. I am tough out with the crew beasting some of them stores in my 'hood. They sellin' to another crew. We sprayed them, killed only one. She talked about my creativity. Fuck that too. She think I'm some dumbshit artist. Fake artist. The fella who do my ink, now he's the artist. Fuckin' good stars on my left hand.

So today when I told her to fuck the list, this bitch don't quit. So I listened. She took one on the list, and then I took one on the list. Fuckin' bitch make me laugh. She be "me" half the time—one alternative is dumbshit training school. She be "me" for that. It her turn. She say, "Training school would be great! No more p.o. beasting you, no hooks." She want us to look at each item and answer a fuckin' question. It sound like school now. But I stay. This time she drag out picture of Michael Jordan—now he's for me. She say to explain to him, not her, about the choices. So we do two—"go back to school" and "prison." Dumb-ass choices, they sound the same. I'll come next week, maybe two. My crew giving me a bad time. I don't tell them I like this bitch. They want to beast her if she give me shit.

SEPTEMBER 15 *People been dissing me all week. Two big fellas in the crew jumped on me for missing the big action this weekend. I was sick and fucking tired and asleep most of the time. They were on my ass and beasting me. I got black eyes and bruised ribs. Dope-pushing assholes. And my momma think I never gonna get the big paper. She want me to find another crew. She don't understand. Belonging to the crew is the only way. Been thinkin' 'bout that tough-ass list the bitch gave me and Michael Jordan. She tol' me to think about ev'ry thing on that dumb-ass list. So I do it when I'm sick. Now what are those piss questions: "Does it get me what I want?" "Can it fuckin' really happen?" "Which bullshit alternative would I like the best?"*

The army. Fuck the army. They don't want me 'cause I can't read too good. And I tell you I ain't working for no $4 a hour. No way. Fraudulent dickheads dissing you all the time. People dissin' you ev'rywhere. School ain't no better. I ain't really been to school since the third, shit, whatever grade. The teachers don't give me no respect. And the work, well it's not so bad. I just not worked in so long. It impossible, tough-ass impossible to catch up. Them punks keep dissing me. No school ain't for me. There just ain't nowhere to go. Of course, I'm not gonna go to juvie. Be smarter on the streets. Juvie be all right for a while, but not for long. It's all right as long as your crew is there. Fuckin' mugs there that are crazy. Some people like the lockup. Not me, man, I like the streets. She say I need to think about others in this fuckin' decision and if my crew is my family. I can't leave them.

She give me a checklist to help decide what to do. This bitch she got me thinking! I never think so much since I was in math when I was little like Mikie. My teacher didn't bullshit. I was good in math. Look at the fuckin' list. Looks like the best "alternative" and be shit is to stay in the crew. And try to miss the hook.

So this bitch she thinks I can make good-ass choices. What a fucking dumbshit thing to say. Of course I can make choices. I already made my choice. She think I die on the streets in some crazy spray. Don't she know I'd rather die on the streets rollin' than in some factory making some little puke-ass part. I ain't gonna get tricked more by some sucker in the system. She know a good program to train me to fix things. Me, a mechanic. That's a big fuckin' joke. When I'm shit I'm gonna own the Benz, not workin' on someone else's.

NOVEMBER 13 *We met together first and talked about my environment. A fuckin' joke. The bitch keep coming up with these questions. Of course I don't need to solve the problem by myself. I've got my crew. If I tried to leave them, they jump on me.*

Then my hard-ass p.o. met with me and my counselor. Parnell's her name. I never knew that before. She was tough in this meeting, and she didn't take no shit from the officer or me. Reminded me of my tough-shit momma. One time momma had a boyfriend who was dissing her and then hit her with a bottle. She be beasting him. He never did come back. We still have some of his shit clothes in the closet. Momma said no use throwing away his only good-ass parts.

She explained what a great job I was doing thinking about my list. And then she explained the risks. We talk about that before, she want to bullshit me about what happen if I be crazy and leave the crew. Last time she fuckin' want to think about risk. I told her no dumbshit "risk." Just a trick! I'm just tryin' to survive!

My p.o. officer, he just shook his head. His puke-faced grin made me mad, and I wanted to jump on him. My crew could wipe the smile off his face. She think I'm cool and really some shit. He is a trouble motherfucker. He want me off probation and into juvie, but I ain't been illing and I ain't done dumbshit. I clean. No dirty bottle. And in one month I'm tricking him 'cause I'm off probation. She looked at me, and I knew not to jump on him. But I wanted to mess his face.

DECEMBER 25   *Christmas is a trick time for the phony men. They be dissing everybody all year long and think they be nice for one day. They ain't real. The mayor promised turkey for everyone who was hungry. What the fuck he think he doin'. People be hungry and eat the bullshit turkey. They starvin' tomorrow. He got his bitches and his dope and his big cars. But I'm not starvin' tomorrow. The hook been on to us and know 'bout paper jobs better than we do. They been dissing us, and some of the crew been illing. They need a fuckin' lesson. The crew is the only thing they got. Look at us here keepin' warm and planning tonight. Down the street we know'd the old fellas running a sure-ass private party. We got lots of mugs in our crew to beast on these motherfuckers. They think they got big juice 'cause they got guns. But we got surprise. Christmas is the best day to show 'em who's in charge of the 'hood.*

CASE QUESTIONS

1. From the perspective of Ms. Parnell, the community counselor, identify Alphonse's problems.

    _____

    _____

    _____

    _____

    _____

    _____

    _____

    _____

2. Describe Alphonse's perspective of his problems.

    _____

    _____

    _____

    _____

    _____

    _____

    _____

    _____

3. List Alphonse's strengths.

_____

_____

_____

_____

_____

_____

_____

4. How do Ms. Parnell's and Alphonse's perspectives differ? How are they similar?

_____

_____

_____

_____

_____

_____

_____

5. List the problems that Alphonse is experiencing and label each as developmental, situational, basic human need, or social change.

_____

_____

_____

_____

_____

_____

_____

6. Describe how Alphonse becomes involved in the human service system.

_____

_____

_____

_____

_____

_____

_____

_____

7. What are the barriers to deliver services to Alphonse?

_____

_____

_____

_____

_____

_____

_____

_____

8. How does Alphonse's gang involvement illustrate characteristics of youth gangs?

_____

_____

_____

_____

_____

_____

_____

EXERCISE: YOU AS THE HUMAN SERVICE PROFESSIONAL

Now that you have an understanding of some basic concepts about those who receive human services and are familiar with Alphonse's case, answer the following questions:

1. Do you think you could work effectively with a client like Alphonse? Why or why not?

_____

_____

_____

_____

_____

_____

_____

_____

2. What do you think are the major challenges you would face if you worked with gangs?

_____

_____

_____

_____

_____

_____

_____

3. Which concepts that describe problems would be most helpful to you in understanding a gang member as an individual who needs human services?

_____

_____

_____

_____

_____

_____

_____

4. How do feel about the language Alphonse uses?

_____

_____

_____

_____

_____

_____

_____

_____

ANOTHER PERSPECTIVE: LIEUTENANT GRACIE JONES

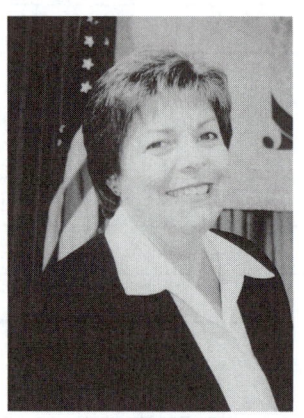

Lieutenant Gracie Jones has more than 25 years experience with a city police department. She initially worked as a patrol officer before being promoted to a criminal investigator and assigned to the narcotics unit. During her career she has handled major crimes such as homicides, rapes, robberies, and assaults as well as all crimes committed by and against juveniles, including child sex abuse, child physical abuse, and missing persons. She created and supervised the gang task force to identify gangs and their members, create educational programs for communities, religious groups, and law enforcement agencies, and intervene in the criminal activities of members.

Lieutenant Jones graduated from college with honors with a degree in sociology. She currently oversees the family protection section of the police department. Specifically, she is responsible for the juvenile unit, domestic violence unit, truancy/curfew center, and the Internet crimes against children task force.

As a police officer, we are trained in the enforcement of law. Our police academy is now 26 weeks long. In that time frame, we are taught everything from state laws, federal laws, how to shoot a firearm, self-defense tactics, defensive driving, policies and procedures, physical fitness, and more. Exactly where does human services fit in this curriculum? How do we train officers to problem solve in the few minutes they have to interact with people? What do we have to offer a streetwise kid like Alphonse? Too often, our job is to arrest people like Alphonse and move on to the next call. So let's see what perspective a police officer might bring to this case.

First, let's look at Alphonse's problems. We must look at his problems from two perspectives: his and his counselor's. Alphonse believes he does not get the respect he deserves from adults and the system. His own mother obviously has her own issues and expects Alphonse to be making money to support her and his little brother. Or so Alphonse believes. What are the real issues in the family? We know

Alphonse doesn't know his father, his mother has been involved with another man who beat her, and she reciprocated. We know through research that 86 percent of all chronic, serious, violent male juveniles come from a home where there is family violence.

Alphonse believes he must belong to the gang to be fed and clothed in style, which will bring him respect from his peers. That stealing, shooting, and committing crimes might land him in "juvie" does not deter him. Neither teachers nor school administrators—with the exception of one teacher—took the time with him in the early years to resolve issues Alphonse faced. He fell behind, which lowered his self-esteem and started his downfall. The third grade seems to be the time in his life where his low self-esteem began. It is the last time he felt good about school and the last time he felt respect from a school official. Alphonse feels his inability to read is what keeps him working the streets instead of pursuing a more viable job. He mentions this when referring to the Army. He is conflicted because he wants the easy money and the extravagant lifestyle but he doesn't want the consequences (jail and longer probation) that might accompany them. He has a probation officer whose only goal, according to Alphonse, is to lock him up.

Intervention at an early age is paramount to keeping kids out of gangs and making them a productive part of society. Alphonse wants off probation but hates the idea that he has to conform to his probation officer's rules and to the rules of the system. You can tell from the way he talks that deep down he would like to get away from the gang, but is afraid of the consequences.

Alphonse's problems from his counselor's perspective aren't that different from his perspective. The difference is that she can be honest about them; he feels he would be viewed as weak to admit them. He hints at several of his problems but admits a couple. The counselor views Alphonse as a child in a man's body. He was pushed into his adulthood too early. She understands why he does not feel respected by society outside his gang. She sees that his inability to read well has hindered his possibility for an honest life. Alphonse has hinted to the counselor that he would get out of his gang if he had the choice, but he would be beaten or killed and would lose the only way he knows for earning money.

Can Alphonse be helped? Of course the answer to that question ultimately rests in his willingness to change. The counselor has found ways into his mind. She showed him respect from the beginning that kept him coming back and having somewhat of an open mind to what she was saying. She may not respect the activities that he participates in, but she respects him as a person and can respect the reasons behind his actions. She does not disrespect him by saying the things he does are wrong. Rather, she looks for alternatives. She makes him look inside himself to see if he has goals that may not be gang-related. She accomplishes this by making it seem more like it comes from him rather than making it seem like an assignment. She also uses the "hero" approach. Making him identify with a hero, in this case Michael Jordan, makes him look at things from a different perspective, not a gang perspective. The fact that one of his heroes is not a gang member gives me the idea that he can have another view and maybe his life is not hopeless.

There are several obstacles that will impede any intervention into this person's life. Alphonse's history with adults and the system makes him wary to trust and believe in anyone. The fact that most of the adults he has come into contact with have been totally authoritative and not supporting furthers this mistrust. He wants rules but not so many that he doesn't have choices. Because of his probation officer's views, he sees the system as merely wanting to get rid of him by incarcerating him or making him adhere to even more rules. All people need rules and even desire them in their life. I have seen this as a reason many youth join gangs. They don't get the structure at home so they find it in the gang. They want rules but still want some freedom of choice unlike school and jail.

Another obstacle is his appearance of weakness especially in front of his brother. He believes he has to be strong and supportive for his brother. He has taught his brother to be self-supportive in case something happens to him and he can no longer take care of him. His educational level and ability is an obstacle but is probably the easiest to tackle. He appears to have the intelligence to learn to read and to gain the knowledge but just needs the motivation to do it.

Probably the biggest obstacle anyone would have in reaching Alphonse is the gang itself. If he attempts to leave, he fears (probably justifiably so) that he would reap a physical beating or death. It is extremely easy to get into a gang but once in, you are their property, and any attempt to leave is taken as a severe insult. This obstacle would probably need the assistance of law enforcement, in which he has no trust. It could also take moving his family, which might be financially impossible. Getting out of the gang will be his responsibility. I have worked with individuals who have expressed a desire to leave but always lack the willpower to stay away. Incarceration and/or probation give them the excuses they need to stay away. His counselor needs to find a way to convince him that leaving the gang is a way of showing strength instead of weakness. The gang has been the only family he could rely on. The counselor would need to incorporate his mother into some sessions and maybe some private sessions in which she would learn how to be a parent and be supportive for her children instead of leaving them to grow up on their own.

The last thing the gang does for him is gives him his means of support. It may be illegal means, but he makes the money he needs to support himself and his brother. Increasing his educational level and ability would help in this endeavor. If someone could direct him into the armed forces, providing his record allows this, he would not only gain a legitimate means of supporting himself, but would also give him the structure he needs in his life. This would also be a possible way to separate him from the gang.

Becoming aware of the reasons our children are doing what they are doing and why they are doing these things is a lifelong study for somebody. The problem is that everything keeps changing. What stays the same is the fact that families are where "it" starts. Both good and bad values are developed in the home. If we don't work to keep families together in a healthy environment, we will continue to lose children to drive-by shootings or prison. The life expectancy of a gang member is 18 to 22 years old. What does society have to offer them after they become an adult? Intervention must begin when the child is first conceived and the family must be nurtured to be healthy and happy. Values and morals must be taught and understood.

EXERCISE: THE LAST WORD

You have the opportunity to have the last word on the terms concepts introduced and the case study presented. Based on what you have learned in this chapter, answer the following questions.

1. When you think about what you have read about human services, what stands out for you?

_____

_____

_____

_____

_____

_____

_____

_____

2. How did the chapter change your ideas and understanding about what human services is?

_____

_____

_____

_____

_____

_____

_____

_____

3. How will you use the information in this chapter in your own life and work?

_____

_____

_____

_____

_____

_____

4. What questions remain unanswered for you?

_____

_____

_____

_____

_____

_____

_____

FOR FURTHER STUDY

BOOKS

Bing, L. (1992). *Do or die*. New York: Perennial. Leon Bing is an investigative reporter who lived with the Bloods and the Crips gangs for four years. He offers an account of life inside a street gang. First-person accounts by the gang members add a realistic quality to the book.

Hagedorn, J. M. (2009). *A world of gangs: Armed young men and gangsta culture*. Minneapolis: University of Minnesota Press. Gangs as a worldwide phenomenon play a significant role in a wide range of activities from drug dealing to extortion to religious and political violence. The author explores gang formation in Chicago, Rio de Janeiro, and Capetown.

Logan, S. (2009). *This is for the Mara Salvatrucha: Inside the MS–13, America's most violent gang*. NY: Hyperion. This is the tale of a street gang that began in Los Angeles in the 1980s and spread across the United States and Central America as experienced by a gang member turned FBI informant.

Savelli, L. (2005). *Gangs across America and their symbols*. Flushing, NY: Looseleaf Law. This pocket guide will help readers to understand the symbols that distinguish members of one gang from another. It focuses on graffiti, dress, hand symbols, body art, and other rituals.

Valentine, B. (2000). *Gangs and their tattoos: Identifying gang members on the street and in prison*. Boulder, CO: Paladin. Written by Bill Valentine who spent 20 years as a correctional officer in Nevada, this book explains in great detail the meaning of tattoos in the gang world. Tattoos represent gang affiliation, gang rank, and values among gang members. Valentine discusses the gang world in prison. In addition, he addresses multicultural issues of African-American, Hispanic, Asian, and Russian gangs.

Venkatesh, S. (2008). *Gang leader for a day: A rogue sociologist takes to the streets*. NY: Penguin. The author writes of his experiences in the 1980s and 1990s as he infiltrated the world of tenant and gang life in Chicago's Robert Taylor Home projects.

MOVIES

West Side Story (1961). Directors: Jerome Robbins and Robert Wise. Starring: Natalie Wood, Richard Beymer, Russ Tamblyn, Rita Moreno. This musical is adapted from Shakespeare's *Romeo and Juliet* and portrays the rivalry between two New York gangs, the Jets and the Sharks.

Boyz N the Hood (1991). Director: John Singleton. Starring: Ice Cube, Cuba Gooding, Jr., Morris Chestnut, Laurence Fishburne. The movie portrays the social problems for black youth growing up in Los Angeles. Three friends take very different paths as they grow up amid violence, drugs, crime, sex, and relationships with parents.

Gangs of New York (2002). Director: Martin Scorsese. Starring: Daniel Day-Lewis, Leonardo DiCaprio, Cameron Diaz. The backdrop for this movie is New York City in the mid-1880s. Gang warfare between well-established immigrants and those new to America dominates an area known as Five Points.

Hustle and Flow (2005). Director: Craig Brewer. Starring: Terence Howard and Anthony Anderson. With help from his friends in the "hood," a pimp tries to break into the music scene in Memphis. He encounters multiple barriers as he tries to escape his life earning money on the streets.

WEB SITES

Explore the Web to learn more about the following:

gangs

street gangs

Gangsorus

Knowgangs.com

developmental

emotional problems

Maslow

social change

social problems

REFERENCES

Curry, G. D., & Decker, S. H. (1998). *Confronting gangs: Crime and community*. Los Angeles: Roxbury.

McKinney, L. (2002). *Instructor's manual for introduction to human services*. Pacific Grove, CA: Brooks/Cole.

Savelli, L. (2005). *Gangs across American and their symbols*. Flushing, NY: Looseleaf Law.

William Gladden Foundation. (1992). *Juvenile gangs*. York, PA: Author.

CHAPTER 6

THE HUMAN SERVICE PROFESSIONAL

The human service professional plays a major role in administering social service programs and providing assistance to clients. The professional uses knowledge, values, and skills to help clients meet their needs. In addition, the professional carries out the goals of the agency he or she represents, assuming a dual commitment to client and agency. The nature of this dual commitment is evident in the field of corrections, focusing on protecting the public as well as rehabilitating clients. To increase your understanding of the work of the human service professional, you will examine the roles and the responsibilities of a corrections officer.

This chapter begins with exercises that encourage you to think about the values and skills discussed in Chapter 6 in your textbook, *Introduction to Human Services, 7th ed.* You will think about human service work, particularly the field of corrections as you complete the exercises. A list of terms and their relevance for human service practice follows. After reading a general description of the field of corrections and specific information about probation and parole, you will be ready to read a firsthand account of a week in the life of a probation officer. Questions to enhance your understanding of professional roles and responsibilities follow as well as a response from a practitioner in the field of corrections. Resources for further study conclude the chapter.

INTRODUCTION

1. Assess the strength of your motivations by indicating your place on the continuum. List additional motivations that you have.

To help others

Strong Motivation .... Little Motivation

To learn more about myself

Strong Motivation .... Little Motivation

Management/administrative opportunities

Strong Motivation .... Little Motivation

Because I was helped by someone

Strong Motivation .... Little Motivation

_____

_____

_____

_____

_____

2. Identify the human service value that would be the most difficult one for you to practice. Why?

_____

_____

_____

_____

_____

3. Which value is the most important for you? Describe how you would use this value to determine your professional actions/behavior.

_____

_____

_____

_____

_____

EXERCISE: WHAT ABOUT YOU?

You learn that an entry-level position is available in corrections working with parolees.

1. Assess the strength of your motivations to work with this client group by indicating your place on the continuum.

To help others

Strong Motivation .... Little Motivation

To learn more about myself

Strong Motivation .... Little Motivation

Management/administrative opportunities

Strong Motivation .... Little Motivation

Because I was helped by someone

Strong Motivation .... Little Motivation

List any other motivations you might have to work in corrections.

_____

_____

_____

_____

2. Identify the human service value that would be most difficult for you to practice if you worked with parolees.

_____

_____

_____

_____

3. Which value do you think would be the most critical in order to be an effective parole officer?

_____

_____

_____

_____

4. What do you believe about people who have been in prison?

I believe

_____

_____

_____

_____

People break laws because

_____

_____

_____

_____

They deserve

_____

_____

_____

_____

When released from prison, they should

_____

_____

_____

_____

KEY IDEAS

The following key ideas will increase your understanding of the human service professional. What motivates a person to pursue a human service career? What do human service professionals believe about helping? What do they actually do?

MOTIVATIONS TO HELP

Individuals choose the profession of human services for a variety of reasons. These reasons include a desire to help others, a need for self-exploration, the desire to be like someone who has helped them, and the goal of administration or management. Motivations for a human service career have both positive and negative aspects. For example, the need to exert control that makes some people effective administrators may also be a need to manipulate or dominate clients. It is important for helpers to understand their motivations and to explore the positive and negative aspects of their attitudes.

VALUES AND PHILOSOPHY

Helpers strive to assist others in need. Within the framework of this work, professionals need to have values that support building rapport and trust with the client. The value of acceptance means being receptive to the client in spite of outward presentation or actions. Tolerance is being open and fair without making judgments. Another value, individuality, means that the helper has positive regard for the uniqueness of each client. Respecting the client's ability to make his or her own decisions demonstrates a respect for the client's right to self-determination. Confidentiality is the helper's assurance to the client that their interactions will remain between the two of them. It is important for all helping professionals to assess their attitudes and values toward their clients and work to uphold these five values.

The foundation for a helping philosophy is based on these values. It includes beliefs about the goodness of human nature, the ways in which individuals grow and develop, and their potential for change.

Helper Characteristics

A number of traits or characteristics contribute to effective helping. These characteristics are self-awareness, the ability to communicate, empathy, and professional commitment. Because the basis of helping is trust and rapport, personal characteristics, not just professional characteristics, are important.

Typology of Human Service Professionals

We can categorize human service providers in three ways; all are based on the individual's level of training or education and competence. Professionals with advanced degrees are specialists in fields such as medicine, psychology, and social work. Human service professionals have a generalist orientation and work with both professionals and nonprofessionals such as volunteers or peer helpers. Nonprofessionals (volunteers and peer helpers) constitute the third category.

Human Service Roles: Direct Service

Immediate and frontline work with clients describes the direct service role. Providing direct service means helpers work face-to-face with individuals, families, and groups to solve their most pressing and serious problems. Professionals act as behavior changers, caregivers, communicators, crisis interveners, empowerers, and teachers.

Human Service Roles: Performing Administrative Work

Many individuals working in human services consider their primary responsibility as oversight and management of services. They may also provide direct care and much of their administrative work relates to supporting the client. These administrative responsibilities include brokering, managing data, evaluating, facilitating services, planning, report writing, developing grant proposals, and allocating resources.

Human Service Roles: Working with the Community

One important component of human service practice is accomplished in the community. Much of this work encompasses advocacy or acting or speaking on behalf of clients. Community work is closely associated with other workers, agencies, client families, neighborhoods, and local, state, and national governments. Possible roles include working as an advocate, community and service networker, community planner, consultant, mobilizer, and outreach worker.

Frontline Worker

This type of worker provides direct service to the client. Most times it means working with the client in the office or agency setting and perhaps in their home as well. Communication, problem solving, and meeting specific outcomes characterize this type of work. A frontline worker establishes a relationship with the client and provides assistance and advocacy.

EXERCISE: YOU AND CORRECTIONS

Assume you are hired by the Department of Corrections to work with parolees. Write a job description of this position. You might think about qualifications, roles, and responsibilities; the services you will provide; and the other professionals/agencies with whom you will work.

_____

_____

_____

_____

_____

_____

_____

_____

FOCUS: CORRECTIONS

The field of **criminal justice** includes three major integrated branches: law enforcement, the courts, and corrections. Law enforcement is focused on the "prevention, investigation, apprehension, or detention of individuals suspected or convicted of offenses against the criminal laws" (Lectric Law Library Lexicon, n.d.). The courts assume responsibility to resolve disputes regarding constitutional, statutory, and common law, and make decisions with the guarantee of due process and equal protection of the law. Criminal cases include those against persons who commit crimes, which are considered offenses against society. The violators are called _offenders_.

Corrections represents a response to offenders who exhibit illegal behaviors. In the United States, several approaches or models have guided the corrections system. Three models are punishment, treatment, and prevention (Allen, Latessa, & Ponder, 2009; Clear, Cole, & Reisig, 2010). The punishment model is based on the concept of retribution; the offender has committed an offense against society and deserves to be punished. Incarceration and capital punishment are two forms of punishment. Some experts believe that strong punishment helps deter future criminal behavior, and that once punished, the offender and other potential offenders will change their behaviors.

A second model focuses on treatment and also advocates a change of behavior for the offender, but recommends programs that assist this change. This model assumes that offenders are troubled and that, with help, they can make positive contributions to society. Although treatment programs do not pamper offenders and do hold them accountable, treatment programs offer education, vocational training, and substance abuse and mental health programs. Treatment programs vary, but the primary goal is to increase the quality of life whether the offender is in prison or living in the community under probation or parole supervision.

The third model to corrections focuses on prevention. Goals for prevention relate to both the individual and the environment. Targeting young children with discipline problems, many prevention programs begin with early intervention with school-age children and their families. For older students, prevention programs include alternatives to punishment such as in-school suspension and community service rather than expulsion. Treatment and prevention programs were developed because the punishment model often did not work and offenders continued to commit crimes (Cole, Gertz, & Bunger, 2003).

Community corrections combines treatment and prevention models in order to meet four major goals: (1) decrease the number of offenders serving in maximum security prisons; (2) provide alternatives to incarceration; (3) reduce financial expenditures within corrections; and (4) develop multiple community programs (SAMAHA, 2005). Under the model of community corrections, offenders receive services and are supervised while residing outside of prison. Diversion, restitution, probation, parole, and halfway houses represent programs within the community framework. The staff working in community corrections settings often have two goals that may appear to be mutually exclusive (Cole, Gertz, & Bunger, 2003). These professionals must uphold the terms of the criminal sentencing, as well as work with offenders to solve problems and become productive citizens. A more detailed discussion of two community corrections programs, probation and parole, follows.

Probation is the largest subsystem of the corrections system. This work first began in 1841 in Boston, Massachusetts, when John Augustus asked a judge to allow him to supervise convicts rather than send them to prison. He supervised adults as well as children. He helped the offenders find jobs and housing, and he conducted an assessment, or social history, which culminated in regular reports to the courts. This type of supervision expanded in the state of Massachusetts, and most states had adopted the probation model by the 1920s (Stephenson-Lang, 2002).

Today, the probation officer works in one of the approximately 2,000 probation agencies with offenders who have committed a crime and are living under supervision in the community rather than in prison. In reality, probation and the promise of good behavior is substituted for prison. While on probation, the offender's activities are restricted according to the terms the judge establishes. The conditions and terms of the probation include length of time, specific requirements such as community service or victim restitution, and potential to re-sentence if offenders violate probation. The probation process includes three separate but integrated action areas, with the probation officer being the center of the activity. The probationer reports regularly to the probation officer, the probation officer *and* other human service professionals who provide treatment and special programs to meet the offender's needs, and the probation officer who supervises and files regular reports to the courts outlining the activities of the probationer. The probation officer's primary responsibility is to ensure the terms of restriction are met and to report to the courts when the terms are violated (Cole, Gertz, & Bunger, 2003).

The probation officer also functions as a caseworker, which means the officer identifies client needs and develops a treatment plan. In reality, many officers do not have the time to work intensely with each client, so they act as brokers and refer clients to agencies within the community.

Just as probation results in supervision prior to incarceration, parole represents supervision after incarceration. The word *parole* derives from the French meaning *to give one's word*, and within the corrections context, it means the offender promises to follow the laws when released from prison. Two individuals developed the concept and the responsibility of parole: Alexander Maconochie, who administered a penal colony off the coast of Australia in the 1840s, and Sir Walter Crofton, who directed Irish prisons in the 1850s. Both Maconochie and Crofton developed penal systems that allowed the practice of early release for good behavior coupled with community supervision. After Zebulon Brockway studied these two models, he implemented a similar system in Elmira, New York, in 1876 (Abadinsky, 1997).

Parole is a way to leave prison and occurs when individuals are released from prison under the supervision of a corrections officer. Today, parole occurs in one of two ways: as a follow-up supervision after an offender has served his or her sentence or as a discretionary decision when an individual is released from prison but has not served the sentence. Since parole follows incarceration, parole officers maintain very strict guidelines for parolees. Rules and conditions of parole include reporting regularly to the parole officer, gaining employment and reporting for work, remaining in the state or local community, maintaining the established curfew, and reporting any arrests or involvement with law enforcement. Violating any of the conditions of parole established by the courts can revoke parole.

There have been several innovations in probation and parole supervision. House arrest as an alternative to imprisonment allows the offenders to live in the community within a tight security network. Where and when he or she leaves home is limited to work, job, and social service or community service programs. Electronic monitoring provides surveillance over offenders who are considered at risk for flight or criminal activity. Some states use it for those on house arrest. Intensive supervised probation or parole represents frequent interaction with the corrections officer and an increased reporting to the courts. Those in intensive supervision programs see their officers once a week, receive visits in their homes, and report the slightest change of their schedule or activities. This supervision also includes curfew, drug testing, community service, and other court-established terms.

The *Occupational Outlook Handbook 2010–11 Edition* describes the probation officer and correctional treatment specialist in the following way:

> Many people who are convicted of crimes are placed on probation instead of being sent to prison. People who have served time in prison are often released on parole. During probation and parole, offenders must stay out of trouble and meet various other requirements. Probation officers, parole officers, and correctional treatment specialists work with and monitor offenders to prevent them from committing new crimes.
>
> *Probation officers*, who are often called *community supervision officers* in some states, supervise people who have been placed on probation. *Correctional treatment specialists*, who may also be known as *case managers* or *correctional counselors*, counsel offenders and create rehabilitation plans for them to follow when they are no longer in prison or on parole. *Parole officers* perform many of the same duties that probation officers perform. The difference is that parole officers supervise offenders who have been released from prison, whereas probation officers work with those who are sentenced to probation instead of parole.

The number of cases a probation officer or correctional treatment specialist handles at one time depends on the needs of offenders and the risks they pose. Higher risk offenders and those who need more counseling usually command more of the officer's time and resources. Caseload size also varies by agency jurisdiction. Consequently, officers may handle from 20 to more than 100 active cases at a time.

Computers, telephones, and fax machines enable the officers to handle the caseload. Probation officers may telecommute from their homes. Other technological advancements, such as electronic monitoring devices, reporting kiosks, and drug screening, also assist probation officers and correctional treatment specialists in supervising and counseling offenders.

Probation officers and correctional treatment specialists work with criminal offenders, some of who may be dangerous. While supervising offenders, they usually interact with many other individuals, such as family members and friends of their clients, who may be angry, upset, or difficult to work with. Workers may be assigned to fieldwork in high-crime areas or in institutions where there is a risk of violence or communicable disease.

Probation officers and treatment specialists are required to meet many court-imposed deadlines, which contribute to heavy workloads. In addition, extensive travel and fieldwork may be required to meet with offenders who are on probation or parole. Workers may be required to carry a firearm or other weapon for protection. They also may be required to collect and transport urine samples of offenders for drug testing. All of these factors make for a stressful work environment. Although the high stress levels can make these jobs very difficult at times, this work also can be very rewarding. Many workers obtain personal satisfaction from counseling members of their community and helping them become productive citizens (U.S. Department of Labor, 2010).

Let's read about a probation officer who works in an intensive supervision program.

CASE STUDY: MEET ALLISON

Allison is a Probation Officer 3 for the state board of probation and parole. This section will describe Allison's work. Then, we will follow her through a typical week as she fulfills her responsibilities as a probation officer. Her position is unusual in that she works on the enhanced supervision level—a more intensive program than traditional probation. In Allison's program, an offender must report to her a minimum of four times a month. She conducts random home visits and curfew checks in the evenings. It is a demanding job and one that others do not want because of the evening work. Yet Allison's caseload is smaller (25–30 cases), and she has a slightly higher salary. A regular caseload is 80–90 cases with contact once a month. First, let's examine the requirements for a probation officer at this level.

MINIMUM QUALIFICATIONS

Education and Experience: Graduation from an accredited college or university with a bachelor's degree and experience equivalent to three years of full-time professional level experience in one or more of the following: probation/parole, counseling, social work, investigative, or legal experience.

Substitution of Experience for Education: Qualifying full-time professional experience may be substituted for the required education, on a year-for-year basis, to a maximum of four years.

Substitution of Education for Experience: Graduate course work credit received from an accredited college or university in social science, behavioral science, criminal justice, criminology, social work, and/or law may substitute for the required experience to a maximum of two years (e.g., an additional 36 graduate quarter hours in one or a combination of the above listed fields may substitute for one year of the required experience).

Necessary Special Qualifications: A valid motor vehicle operator's license may be required.

Examination Method: Education and Experience, 100% for Career Service positions.

Allison has a bachelor's degree in human services and had previously worked as a county probation officer before she applied for this state position. When she did apply, she was given credit for her field experience in human services, making it possible for her to begin her job as a Probation Officer 2. After a year, she applied for a job as a Probation Officer 3. Now, let's consider the written job description as published by the personnel department.

EXAMPLE OF DUTIES AND RESPONSIBILITIES

1. Leads others in the supervision of a caseload of offenders; advises and consults with probation and/or parole officers of lower classification on individual offender cases; offers recommendations on techniques and methods to handle problem areas; may supervise a caseload of offenders; may supervise a small staff.
2. Leads or supervises others in a variety of investigations; gathers evidence on offenders for disposition by the court; collects prior arrest and conviction information from court files, prior institutional files, law enforcement records, telecommunications networks and other states; gathers information from offenders, defendants, witnesses, victims, and family members through on-site visits; compares legal standards against factual information collected as a result of the investigations in order to provide the court or board with recommendations for feasible dispositions or for agency decisions regarding security, treatment, or supervision of offenders.
3. Leads or supervises others in evaluating offender's adjustment to the community; directs the offender to treatment, educational, or vocational referral agencies; establishes a supervision schedule for offenders according to needs and risk assessment instruments; follows up on the offender's adjustment by making periodic visitations or telephone contacts to the residence, place of employment, school, family, or treatment agencies.
4. Conducts fact-finding investigations to prosecute violators; handles special court and board requests, or gathers factual information to place inmates on parole; recommends that a violation warrant or subpoena be issued.

5. May collect facts gathered from witnesses, victims, arresting officer's reports, and district attorney's files, which help the court or board determine if the offender can remain in the community; recommends that an offender violation warrant or subpoena be issued, or that the offender be kept under supervision, based on the evidence at hand.

6. Ensures accuracy and thoroughness of reports of subordinates; may check reports or case files; may identify and discuss corrective action needed with the probation/parole officer to ensure compliance with agency policy.

7. Enters chronological contacts of the parole investigation process; discusses corrective action needed with the probation/parole officer manager to ensure compliance with agency policy; identifies criminal activities and background information in reports or standard forms requested by the parole board.

8. Represents the organization in a variety of formal and informal public contacts; exchanges information with representatives of local mental health centers, rehabilitation and employment services, and other community agencies about programs that can help the offender adjust to the community; gives talks to civic organizations and schools to provide information about probation and parole services.

9. May provide casework services and oversees office operations; assists district supervision by handling technical case problems and managing office operations in the absence of the supervisor; may supervise a small staff; may develop job plans, conduct interim interviews, and annual performance evaluations.

10. May attend parole board meetings and/or hearings; participates in inquiry revocation hearings to state circumstances of offenders' parole activities and violations; prepares records and other information for the board in order to expedite review of cases.

11. Participates in training and/or delivery of such specialized programs as intensive supervision, GED, employment counseling, and alcohol and drug abuse treatment counseling; attends a prescribed pre-service and in-service training to learn policies and procedures.

12. Uses an automobile for field contacts with offenders as well as their families, employers, schools, law enforcement officials, and community assistance agencies.

13. May be required to perform urinalysis screens on offenders; uses electronic monitoring equipment and a personal computer.

Now, you will read the diary that Allison kept for a week she describes as typical for her. We will see how it compares with the official duties and responsibilities listed in the job description. Her week begins on Sunday.

THE CASE

SUNDAY, 6:00 P.M.–11:00 P.M. *My week began with a scheduled monthly "ride along" with the police department. "Ride along" refers to times when both the police officer and the probation/parole officer are doing curfew checks on offenders, as well as other service calls to which the police officer may respond during the shift. This participation is a collaborative effort for Community Policing. All offenders on the Enhanced Supervision Program (this is my program) have a 6:00 P.M.–6:00 A.M. curfew unless the probation officer has given permission otherwise. Because of limited police department staffing, I'm not able to take an officer on every home contact so when I do a "ride along," I try to see those offenders who need a police officer at their home. This could be someone who has not been home on their curfew checks the past time or two, and I'm in the process of deciding if the offender needs to wear an ankle bracelet. In my job I have the option of putting people on electronic monitoring if they're not adhering to the curfew. Or perhaps we visit someone who is not working or perhaps their probation isn't going well. I let these folks know that the police know where they live and the police can come by any time with or without me.*

On this particular Sunday, I was able to do a couple of my checks. I "ride along" once a month regardless of whether we do any curfew checks. It is a way to get to know the officers. And it also provides an opportunity for me to point out where someone lives and to ask that the officer keep an eye out.

Let me explain about curfews because this is an important part of enhanced probation. Curfew is 6:00 P.M. for everyone on enhanced probation. They must have permission from me to deviate from curfew. If they have a night job and we know their hours, then we can give specific permission to attend. If they are in drug treatment that requires meetings after 6:00 P.M., then they can call and get permission for that. We're not going to stop someone from getting treatment or working. But often an offender calls about going to a 7:00 P.M. movie—no permission for that! What this means though, in terms of my work, is that I have a cellular phone with me at all times. I can be reached in or out of the office at any time so there is no reason why an offender can't request permission. When I get a call, then I must document it in case notes. We are now set up to do this from home so I don't have to wait to get into the office to make these notes.

MONDAY, 10:00 A.M.–4:30 P.M. *On Mondays I usually work in the office and today was no exception. Generally, Mondays are devoted to paperwork, preparing Violation of Probation warrants/reports and any orders needed for the court. At 2:00 P.M., all new offenders who have been referred to the Enhanced Supervision Program by the court report to the office to meet with my supervisor and the Community Corrections Program manager from the police department. This referral is the result of a pre-sentence investigation that is prepared for the court. It includes information about the offender's physical data, prior criminal record, education, health, family, employment, and finances. Based on this report, the offender is considered high, medium, or low risk regarding the probability of making it on probation. If a person is deemed high risk, then that individual is placed in the Enhanced Supervision Program.*

High risk includes anyone who has been on probation before and had his or her probation revoked. Offenders get several chances at probation. You would think that if they didn't do it right the first time that they would be incarcerated but that's not the way it happens. If someone has an unstable living situation, they may end up on enhanced. We might also move them to a halfway house. A lengthy criminal history would also qualify an individual for the enhanced program. This program is an alternative to prison and we try to work with them for a minimum of six months.

If they do everything they need to do during the six-month period—report in every week, pay court costs, make restitution, go through drug and alcohol treatment, not violate curfew, and pick up no new charges—then they may be reevaluated and move to regular probation. I haven't had many do that. On the other hand, if the enhanced probation doesn't work, then the probation is revoked and the offender must serve the sentence. In reality, it's cheaper to keep an offender in the community than prison so we do what we can to make enhanced supervision work.

All Probation Officer 3s assist in the Monday afternoon meeting. There are a number of agenda items that require all staff to participate:

1. **Discuss all conditions of supervision.** *Obeying the laws of the United States, not picking up any new charges, being employed, receiving permission to travel, immediately reporting all arrests, and carrying their ID cards with them at all times are examples of conditions.*
2. **Sign necessary paperwork.** *Originals go in our files and offenders get copies of everything. We get their signatures on all forms.*
3. **Take digital photos of each offender.** *The photos are then e-mailed to the police department to a computer data bank so the police are able to pull up an offender's picture and any information they need about name, address, and charges. On a "ride along," a police officer with a laptop computer can pull up this data bank, and I can find my probationers as the officer scrolls through the data bank.*
4. **Conduct a drug screen on each offender.** *If we find someone who isn't clean, we have to get them in some kind of treatment. A clean drug screen is the best finding. Policy is to do a drug screen every three months, but we often do more than [that]. Sometimes these happen in the office, sometimes at home, sometimes at work. It's important that the drug screens are random. For example, if offenders know drug screens occur on Tuesdays and that cocaine stays in the system two–three days, then they won't use past Saturday.*
5. **Assign offender to a probation/parole officer.** *This assignment depends on where an offender resides. Each probation/parole officer works a certain district or area of the county.*
6. **Explain Community Policing and inform offenders that a police officer may come to their home periodically to check on them.**

All of this takes about an hour and a half. As the supervisor talks with the offenders, staff are taking the digital photos. Then, the drug screen happens. Finally, all felons are then referred to the health department because in this state, they have to submit a DNA sample. Many times this happens in the prison, so if we have an offender who has done any considerable amount of time before, then their DNA is already on file.

Mondays are busy!

TUESDAY, 7:00 A.M.–5:30 P.M. *Each probation/parole officer determines his or her reporting schedule. These are the days and times that are set aside for offenders to see their probation officers. My reporting day is Tuesday and I see offenders all day. During these meetings offenders report any changes that have occurred. Each offender is required to report at least four times a month to provide employment verification and proof of payments made on court costs/restitution and supervision fees. At this time we also check the status of any special conditions that may have been court-ordered. These conditions may include community service, drug/alcohol treatment programs, and vocational training. Drug screens may also be administered during the visit.*

Today was nonstop chaos because I saw offenders from 7:00 A.M. until 5:30 P.M. Because I see these folks once a week and I visit them in their homes and at work, I actually see them more than friends and family. I know what's going on with them. When they come in each week, it may be that nothing has changed since last Tuesday or the night before when I was at their house. This means the office visit is not as long as you might think it would be, although the first time I meet with offenders does take more time because I review backgrounds and their files.

The chaos comes from trying to see everyone. Some people want to come before work and we try to accommodate them so I try to begin at 7:00 A.M. I actually have a group of people who show up because they have to be at work at 8:00 A.M. I'm not a morning person so it's a challenge for me. I'm here all day and I don't leave.

Wednesday, 10:00 A.M.–4:30 P.M. *Today I worked in the office, reviewing new cases that I received on Monday and making sure things are in order. Once all the paperwork was completed, I took some warrants and reports to the Criminal Court Clerk's office. A warrant states any violations by the offender, has my signature, and then goes to the judge for his or her signature. I have never had a judge refuse to sign a warrant. The judges in this area work well with us. In fact, some of the judges I work with now are the same ones I worked with in county probation. You build trust with judges so they know you're not bringing a warrant to them that is inaccurate or questionable. Accompanying the warrant is a violation report that provides general information about the offender and lists the violations that have occurred. We can also include recommendations that the judge may or may not accept. For example, should probation be revoked? Or a request to let us continue to work with the offender a few more months, get him or her into treatment, or move the offender to a halfway house.*

I finished the day making sure all my contact notes had been entered into the system. Our case notes are computerized and it is important that they are current. This information is important to the court, probation officers, and the police.

Thursday, 8:30 A.M.–5:30 P.M. *I worked in the office until a Drug Court staffing at 3:30 P.M. This is a meeting of Drug Court counselors, the judge, and anyone else who is working with an offender. Participating in Drug Court is one of those special conditions that the judge can mandate for an offender who is addicted to drugs, alcohol, or both. The 9-to-18-month program is a drug intervention treatment program designed to provide a cost-effective alternative to traditional criminal case processing. It is a strenuous program, and it is difficult for offenders to get through it. Two officers from this office attend each week. I now have an offender on my caseload who is participating in Drug Court, which is why I attended today. The staffing part occurs from 3:30 P.M. to 4:30 P.M. and is led by the judge who asks for updates on all offenders in the program. The actual Drug Court occurs from 4:30 P.M. until 5:30 P.M. The judge sits behind a bench but doesn't wear a robe and there's no district attorney present. It's fairly casual. Each offender comes up individually to the bench and talks with the judge. If they've done something they weren't supposed to do, then sanctions are administered. The sanctions depend on the violation. For example, if someone fails a drug screen, the judge may sentence him or her to a weekend in jail.*

So I ended my day at Drug Court.

FRIDAY, 7:30 A.M.–11:30 A.M. *I reported to the County Criminal Court Division III this morning. Two offenders were on the docket today. One was a status check for restitution payment and overall progress. To this point, the offender has been doing well—all court costs/restitution paid in full, supervision fees current, employed, no positive drug screens, and no curfew violations. I asked that the offender be taken off any further docket and, if any problems arise, I will notify the court.*

A revocation of probation hearing was also set for today. The offender has been in custody for approximately a month on a Violation of Probation warrant. He was participating in an intensive outpatient program and tested positive for the use of marijuana. He also has not maintained full-time employment for one month. After the offender consulted with his attorney, he determined it was in his best interest to submit to the revocation of probation. The offender will be given credit for any time he has been in custody before being transported to the Department of Corrections. Had he decided not to submit to the revocation, a hearing would have been held. At that time I would have been called to testify to the violations that have occurred and possibly the offender would be called to testify. If necessary, other people may be called to testify (other probation/parole officers, police officers, etc.).

CASE QUESTIONS

1. How accurately does the written job description reflect the realities of the job Allison has?

    _____

    _____

    _____

    _____

    _____

    _____

    _____

2. Describe the role of technology in facilitating Allison's work.

    _____

    _____

_____

_____

_____

_____

_____

_____

3. Based on what you have read in Allison's diary, identify the human service values that she practices in her work.

_____

_____

_____

_____

_____

_____

_____

4. How does Allison describe the challenges in a typical week?

_____

_____

_____

_____

_____

_____

_____

5. How does Allison embody the characteristics of an effective helper?

_____

_____

_____

_____

6. Where does Allison fit in the typology of helping professionals and why?

7. List situations that illustrate her interactions with other professionals.

8. How are the major categories of human service responsibilities (direct service, administration, and community work) illustrated in both the written job description and Allison's diary?

9. How does Allison fit the description of a frontline worker?

_____

_____

_____

_____

_____

_____

_____

EXERCISE: YOU AS THE HUMAN SERVICE PROFESSIONAL

Now that you have a basic understanding of the probation/parole system, answer the following questions:

1. What is your reaction to Allison's week?

_____

_____

_____

_____

_____

_____

_____

2. Compare the job description you wrote in an earlier exercise with Allison's job description.

_____

_____

_____

_____

_____

_____

3. What do you think are the challenges of working with offenders?

_____

_____

_____

_____

_____

_____

_____

4. Identify any concerns you might have about visiting an offender at home.

_____

_____

_____

_____

_____

_____

_____

5. In your opinion, how can society effectively deal with offenders?

_____

_____

_____

_____

_____

_____

_____

6. What qualities or characteristics do you have that would help you work effectively with offenders?

_____

_____

_____

_____

_____

_____

_____

_____

7. Describe the difficulties you would encounter.

_____

_____

_____

_____

_____

_____

_____

ANOTHER PERSPECTIVE: CARL PAPA, JR.

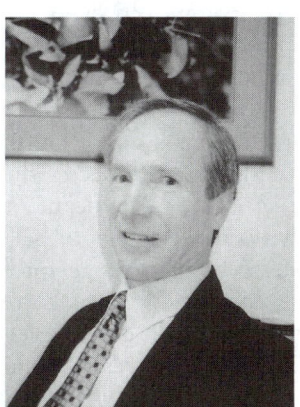

Carl Papa, Jr., has 30 years experience in the field of corrections, having served at both state and federal levels. For three years he served as a state probation/parole officer before serving in various positions in the federal court system for 27 years, 10 of which he served as the Chief of United States Pretrial Services in the Eastern District of Tennessee. As a Chief of Pretrial Services, hey supervised a staff of 17 in three cities. Chief Papa has a bachelor's degree in psychology and sociology and a master's degree in educational psychology. He enjoys scuba diving, snow skiing, and taking long trips throughout the United States on his Harley-Davidson motorcycle all activities he is enjoying in retirement.

My initial impression of Allison's week-long diary is that she works extremely hard. She has a full schedule working some days until 10:00 at night. Having served as a state/federal probation and pretrial services officer, I'm familiar with different types of supervision of defendants/offenders in the field of corrections as well as with general caseloads and intensive caseloads. Intensive caseloads are mostly drug cases. These individuals must be seen frequently (usually at least one time per week) to make sure they have not reverted back to drug use. Other individuals on an intensive caseload are a danger to the community or a specific person and you need to know the individual's whereabouts. This may be accomplished through an electronic monitoring program or through home confinement restrictions. It's labor intensive and it can wear you out keeping up with these individuals. I can see someone in Allison's position getting burned out in that job. It sounds like she is doing a heck of a job keeping up with it all.

People choose a career in corrections for several reasons. First, it's interesting dealing with people who have violated the law. I don't know why that is, but it is intriguing. Just like it is interesting for me to go to Sturgis, South Dakota, to the Harley motorcycle rally. In corrections, you are exposed to people from all walks of life—people who have lived different lifestyles from you and have different values. Some of their lifestyles and behaviors are foreign to mainstream society. Second, a career in corrections allows you to help people. That's part of your personality. When you work closely with someone like an offender, you get to know that person so well—who they are, where they live, with whom they live, what work they do. You go to their homes and meet their families. You learn about their problems (marital, financial, whatever the case) and you do what you can to help them. You broker the services they need to help reduce their risk of re-offending. This is one of the major components of the correctional system.

Another component of corrections is protection of the community. For example, when a person is arrested, we do a background investigation and submit a report to the judge. We make a recommendation to the judge whether the person is a danger to the community and whether he or she should be released on a bond. We may recommend conditions of release to protect the community and to assist the person while on bond. For example, as a condition of release there may be drug screens on the person in a drug case or with drug history or may have employment ordered as a condition if the individual is unemployed. Many cases might have a condition of release that require monitoring their associations with other individuals or groups, because it may involve organized crime or gang activity, which becomes a problem for the community.

Electronic monitoring may be implemented as a condition to help us know an individual's whereabouts. Home visits are also used to access the defendant's compliance, which may include talking to a spouse or significant other to get a good picture of what is taking place. You may do other things to help; for example, assist the individual with upgrading employment or arrange for mental health/substance abuse counseling. However, whatever the conditions of release, if there is a violation of the law or the conditions that are ordered, then we protect the community through independent investigation, possibly having the person picked up and returned to jail until there is a hearing before a judge. Protection of the community always comes first and that is when interesting investigation techniques come into play.

Enhanced supervision is intensive and it works. It's hard to get into trouble if there's someone looking over your shoulder monitoring your every move. I have helped individuals avoid some previous associations or fall back into bad habits that led them to their trouble in the first place. It's a hard thing to do though. Some pretrial offices, Miami, for instance, have an enhanced unit. These officers come to work at 7:00 or 8:00 at night and they go into the community, stopping by homes, making sure these gang members are where they need to be, and conducting drug tests in the middle of the night. Allison's job is dangerous. However, the amount of time you invest in an individual's case can make a difference in that person's life. Most defendants or offenders are doing better after supervision than they were before coming into the criminal justice system. Success in this job is measured in different ways, and for those on enhanced supervision, not being arrested in six months can be success.

There are a variety of job duties that keep probation and parole officers interested in their jobs. Caseloads and requirements of the cases are changing constantly. Offenders are getting off of supervision, as new ones come onto your caseload. You never know what your day in this job may hold. This is true in my work at Pretrial Services. Someone robs a bank at noon, by 2:00 P.M. they may be in custody in a lockup, and by 4:00 P.M. pretrial has jumped into action. So, there is excitement. Some people, however, don't like unpredictability. They like to go to work and know they have a stack of papers they need to move from the in-box to the out-box in the allotted eight hours. Tomorrow they're going to have another stack of papers and nothing interrupts that daily flow.

Allison might be working on a project when someone on her caseload gets arrested. That's more work for her because she has to gather arrest reports, interview her client and others involved, then decide what she's going to recommend to the judge. Should this person be given another chance, or has he truly violated the conditions of probation or parole? Does his release need to be revoked? The same is true in pretrial. We may be helping someone, perhaps assisting their family as more of a counselor, when a crisis with another case arises. You must have the ability to change from a counselor to almost that of a prosecutor. If someone violates a condition of release, it takes priority. But, while you are attempting to deal with that case, you get a call that new arrests are on their way to you, and they now take priority. I think this keeps the job interesting, because it keeps changing.

Corrections is also an opportunity to be aware of changing crimes. For example, ten years ago, cocaine and marijuana were the drugs of choice. Before we knew it, crack cocaine became very popular, and we couldn't keep up with the supervision of these cases, because the drug was so addictive. Three years later, methamphetamine became the drug of choice. Last summer not only were we dealing with the local manufacturing of methamphetamine, but we had Mexicans dealing pure Mexican methamphetamine in this area. We've never had this problem before. We've had illegal aliens from Mexico and other countries working on farms. We'd round them up under immigration laws and send them back home, which was a revolving door as they would soon return. But now we have Mexicans who have rented farms and are dealing methamphetamine or cocaine. They have become very organized groups with lookouts and surveillance equipment. It's a new challenge for us, especially when they do not speak English. We must locate Spanish interpreters and even try to locate lawyers who speak some Spanish. Other agencies such as the Drug Enforcement Administration, Immigrations Services, and the U.S. Marshal Service are involved with us, so it gets a bit wild. But it's interesting, and there is always a new challenge to encounter.

You ask what qualities make a good probation or parole officer? When I interviewed someone for a job in my district, I looked for a person who has some experience dealing with a caseload or counseling with people. Frequently, police officers or lawyers will apply for these federal positions in field supervision. In many cases, they have the wrong kind of training. We want someone who is open-minded. I needed people who can consider several factors before acting. First, people are innocent until proven guilty. Second, we have to be able to continually evaluate danger to the community. Third, risk of flight (nonappearance) is another consideration my officers must evaluate. Sometimes, we have to recommend a bond because the person is innocent until proven guilty and there exist conditions of release that can be imposed and that the person can meet. This can be a difficult decision depending on the specific offense charged. For example, we have an influx of cyber crimes, especially Internet pornography. The individual charged with this type of an offense may still be entitled to a bond, regardless of how we feel about the crime. Keeping the community safe from this type of offender is extremely difficult. In today's society, how do you keep someone off the Internet, or away from children?

Many of the officers in the federal system came from the state system like I did. I did pre-sentence reports, background investigations, managed different types of caseloads, and have continually dealt with police officers, attorneys, and judges in the process. I maintained records on my cases, which were subject to examination, so I had to clearly reflect what I had done on any given case. I wanted to hire people who have this type of track record in dealing with this type of work. The federal system is often perceived as a step up for someone in the state system. For example, it may be a step up for Allison. This is because most states do not pay as well as the federal government nor do they have as good a retirement package. Some states, however, like California, do pay more. Another challenge is that some of the agencies that are concerned with homeland security such as the Federal Bureau of Investigations (FBI) and the Bureau of Alcohol, Tobacco, and Firearms (ATF) will pay officers more.

Finally, there is an element of danger in this type of work. Some people aren't interested in that; others love it. People who go to the police academy love it. People who work undercover love it even more. If you're looking for excitement and a challenge, if you want to help people, if you want to protect the community, then corrections is a good field. Starting at the county or the state level is a great place to get the experience. This was Allison's route for experience and I think she would agree that it prepared her well.

EXERCISE: THE LAST WORD

You have the opportunity to have the last word on the terms introduced and the diary you read. Based on what you have learned in this chapter, answer the following questions.

1. When you think about what you have read about human services in this chapter, what stands out for you?

_____

_____

_____

_____

_____

---

2. How did the chapter change your ideas and understanding about what human services is?

___

3. How will you use the information in this chapter in your own life and work?

___

4. What questions remain unanswered for you?

FOR FURTHER STUDY

BOOKS

Alarid, L. F., & del Carmen, R. V. (2010). *Community-based corrections*. Belmont, CA: Wadsworth. The array of punishment and treatment programs that are alternatives to prison and jail are the focus of this book.

Cornelius, G. F. (2009). *The art of the con: Avoiding offender manipulation*. Alexandria, VA: American Correctional Association. This book is described as a must-read for new or veteran corrections officers because of its perspective from the criminal mind.

Hess, K. M. (2009). *Criminal investigation*. Belmont, CA: Delmar Cengage Learning. Practical procedures techniques, and applications of private and public investigations provide a foundation for criminal investigation.

Schmalleger, F., & Smkla, J. O. (2000). *Corrections in the 21st century*. New York: McGraw-Hill. This book introduces the ideas and practices characteristic of modern corrections.

Schroeder, D. J., & Lombardo, F. A. (2000). *Corrections officer exam*. Garden Grove, CA: Learning Express. This book prepares applicants for the exam to become a municipal, county, state, federal, or private corrections officer.

MOVIES

Brubaker (1980). *Director: Stuart Rosenberg*. Starring: Robert Redford, Jane Alexander. Redford plays a newly appointed warden who first enters prison posing as an inmate. He begins to make changes at the prison and encounters resistance from his staff. Finally, he is forced to make a choice to "play the game" for a few changes or resign.

Dead Man Walking (1996). *Director: Tim Robbins*. Starring: Susan Sarandon, Sean Penn. The title refers to slang used by prison guards when escorting death row prisoners from their cells to the execution chambers. A nun, while comforting a convicted killer on death row, empathizes with both the killer and the victim's families. The emotional issue of the death penalty is front and center in this movie.

The Green Mile (1999). *Director: Frank Darabont*. Starring: Tom Hanks, David Morse. The focus of this movie is the lives of the guards on death row and their encounter with a black man accused of child murder and rape, who also has the power of faith healing. It is a compelling study of human injustice and charity.

Monster Ball (2002). *Director: Marc Forster*. Starring: Billy Bob Thornton, Halle Berry. After a family tragedy, a racist prison guard reexamines his attitudes while falling in love with the African American wife of the last prisoner he executed.

The Shawshank Redemption (1994). *Director: Frank Darabont*. Starring: Tim Robbins, Morgan Freeman. Andy Dufresne (Tim Robbins) has been convicted of murdering his wife and is sentenced to life imprisonment. The drama is set in the 1940s, portraying the prison life of this young banker. The story focuses on the life of Andy, the relationship between him and his friend Red (Morgan Freeman), and his remarkable escape.

WEB SITES

Explore the Web to learn more about the following:

American Correctional Association

American Probation and Parole Association

incarceration

recidivism

The National Criminal Justice Reference Service

criminal justice

parole

parole officer

probation

probation officer

REFERENCES

Abadinsky, H. (1997). *Probation and parole.* Upper Saddle River, NJ: Simon & Schuster.

Allen, H. E., Latessa, E., & Ponder, B. (2009). *Corrections in America: An introduction* (12th ed.). New York: Macmillan.

Clear, T., Cole, G., & Reisig, M. (2010). *American corrections* (9th ed.). Belmont, CA: Wadsworth.

Cole, G. F., Gertz, M. G., & Bunger, A. (2003). *Criminal justice system: Politics and policies* (8th ed.) Belmont, CA: Wadsworth.

Lectric Law Library Lexicon. (n.d.) *Law enforcement.* Retrieved from http://www.lectlaw.com/def/l008.htm

Samaha, J. (2005). *Criminal justice.* Belmont, CA: Wadsworth.

Stephenson-Lang, J. (October 2002). *Probation in the criminal justice system.* Retrieved from http://cjstudents.com/probation.htm.

U.S. Department of Labor. (2010). *Occupational outlook handbook 2010–11 edition: Probation officers and correctional treatment specialists.* Retrieved from http://www.bls.gov/oco/ocos265.htm.

7 # The Helping Process

The helping relationship is the foundation of the helping process. In fact, many helping professionals consider it more important than the helping strategies used to address client problems. They believe that the skillful application of helping strategies is not very effective unless a helping relationship has been established between the human service professional and the client. This chapter explores the helping process and the concepts that will help you understand this process.

The chapter begins with an activity which will prepare you for thinking about how your cultural background impacts the helping relationship. The second activity requires you to think about the helping process in terms of your own life experience. A list of key concepts and their definitions follows. Knowledge of these terms will help you understand the case of Gloria, a Puerto Rican woman, as she experiences the helping process. An introduction to Puerto Rican culture precedes the presentation of Gloria's case and provides a context for her experiences. Questions that help you apply the concepts discussed follow the case study. Finally, a human service professional offers her perspective on the case and its implications for other helping professionals. Additional resources for further study conclude the chapter.

INTRODUCTION

The purpose of this activity is to provide you with an opportunity to apply concepts introduced in Chapter 7 of *Introduction to Human Services, 7th ed.* We encourage you to begin thinking about the cultural influences in your own life. The first activity focuses on you while the second activity encourages you to examine your environment.

Activity 1

Choose another student in class to talk with about the cultural heritage of your names. Listen as your partner talks about his or her name. Consider cultural factors such as race, ethnicity, and religion that may have influenced the names. Share experiences you have had with your name or feelings you have experienced as a result of your name.

ACTIVITY 2

There are many cultural influences found in the environment in which we live. With your partner, identify both material and non-material things that are present in your community that come from another culture. These items may include possessions, movies, literature, and ideas. Discuss the cultural influences present in your everyday life.

DISCUSSION

After completing these two activities, answer the following questions:

1. How important are names in terms of identities? What is your opinion about the practice of "Americanizing" the names of those who come to the United States to live and/or study?

---

2. Since our names are given to us, is there another name you would select as more representative of you as an individual?

| TABLE 7.1 | CULTURE: THE SILENT PARTNER WORKSHEET |

Aspects of life impacted by culture	Implications for helping professionals
Language	_____
Rituals observed	_____
Perspectives on work and activity	_____
Pace of life—perspectives on relaxing	_____
Celebrating holidays	_____
Expression of emotions	_____
Feelings about life, death, and illness	_____
Definitions of the family and meanings of "family"	_____
Attitudes toward seeking help	_____
Sex role definitions	_____
Meaning of friendship	_____
Perspectives on control of nature	_____
Perspectives on time	_____
Perceptions of individual identity	_____
Approaches to decision making	_____
Nonverbal communication	_____

Worksheet developed by Bea Wehrly, Professor of Counselor Education, 74 Horrabin Hall, Western Illinois University, Macomb, IL 61445

_____

_____

3. What conclusions can you draw about cultural influences?

_____

_____

_____

_____

Table 7.1 is a worksheet to help you think about culture and its implications for helping professionals. A list of cultural aspects are on the left. Describe the impact of each upon the helping process.

EXERCISE: WHAT ABOUT YOU?

Think about a time in your life when you received help from someone else, for example, a friend, a counselor, a minister, your parents, or a teacher. You may describe an experience that was positive or negative. Describe as completely as you can what happened, the helper, your feelings, and the outcome(s).

KEY IDEAS

The helping process is just that—a process. It has a beginning, an end, and a flow that varies from relationship to relationship. A brief discussion of the following important terms will help you understand the helping process.

INITIAL INTERVIEW

This term describes the first face-to-face meeting between the client and the helper. It marks the beginning of the helping process and involves an exchange of information about the client, the problem, the agency, and its services. A primary goal of this meeting is building trust and rapport between the client and helper. Greetings, handshakes, introductions, and conversational icebreakers facilitate this goal.

PROBLEM IDENTIFICATION

Critical to the helping process is exploring and clarifying what is troubling the client. Accurately assessing the difficulty involves seeking answers to questions such as the following: Who is involved? What is the influence of the environment? How does the client experience the problem? Does the helper understand the client's feelings about the situation?

TERMINATION

The end or conclusion of the helping relationship is termination and it happens in both positive and negative ways. The best case scenario occurs when the client reaches the goal and no longer needs assistance from the helper. Other ways that termination occurs include: the helper is promoted or quits; the client moves or simply never shows up again;or the school year ends. In these cases, termination may take place without problem resolution.

COMMUNICATION SKILLS

Communication skills in the helping process allow the helper and the client to engage in a dialogue to explore perceptions, ideas, problems, and concerns. The helper understands the message sent by the client and vice versa; in other words, communication is two-way. Specific skills that facilitate this interaction are listening to both verbal and nonverbal messages, responding verbally and nonverbally, and questioning appropriately. Each of these skills helps the professional establish a relationship with the client.

QUESTIONING

The purpose of this communication skill is to elicit information. Appropriate times to ask a question include beginning an interview ("Could you tell me a little about yourself?"), obtaining specific information ("How long have you been ill?"), and eliciting examples of specific behavior ("What was your reaction to that?"). The skill of questioning is often a challenge to beginning professionals. Too many questions, for example, can cause the client to feel defensive in which case it becomes difficult to maintain rapport.

PARAPHRASING

This term means the restatement of what the client has said by the helper. The helper uses words, phrases, or both that are interchangeable with the client's words. Helpers use this technique to establish rapport by letting the client know that the helper listened well and therefore, understood what was said.

CRISIS

An individual's emotional response to a hazardous or threatening situation defines a crisis. It is not the situation, for example, a rape, a natural disaster like a hurricane or a tornado, or the sudden loss of a loved one, which defines the crisis. It is the individual's interpretation or perception of a situation or of an event. The potential for crisis occurs when pressures or stresses disrupt an individual's equilibrium or balance. The stages of crisis development escalate as the individual's anxiety level increases because of the failure of coping mechanisms or problem-solving abilities. Then, tension and anxiety rise to an unbearable level and the individual experiences a crisis.

CRISIS INTERVENTION

The skills and strategies that a helper uses when faced with a client's crisis are an example of a short-term helping process. Although it occurs at a much faster pace than other helping relationships and is time limited, the helper's role in crisis intervention is similar to that in other helping relationships. In crisis intervention, the helper assesses the situation (identifies the problem), plans an intervention (plan development), and implements the intervention (service delivery). This may mean finding a placement for the client, protecting the client from harming oneself or others, or seeking medical help for the client. Longer-term service delivery is provided from another source, usually a helping professional or an agency to which the client is referred.

Listening and responding are especially important as the helper assesses the client's situation, activates a support network for the client, and helps the client focus on a course of action. Nonverbal, physical gestures such as touch, are powerful tools to aid in the establishment of the helping relationship.

EXERCISE: YOU AND THE HELPING PROCESS

This exercise will expand your thoughts about the helping process. Before you begin, review your description of the help you received in the exercise "What About You?" at the beginning of the chapter. As you think about that experience, respond to the following questions:

1. How did your experience illustrate the initial interview and the termination of the helping process?

_____

_____

_____

_____

_____

_____

_____

_____

2. What communication skills facilitated or hindered the development of the relationship?

_____

_____

_____

_____

_____

_____

_____

3. Describe how the helper used questions in your situation.

_____

_____

_____

_____

_____

_____

_____

_____

4. What did the helper do that you liked or disliked?

_____

_____

_____

_____

_____

_____

_____

5. As you think about crisis intervention, was your problem a crisis? If not, how might it have become a crisis?

_____

_____

_____

_____

_____

_____

_____

_____

FOCUS: PUERTO RICAN CULTURE

The demographic shifts now occurring in the population of the United States make it more ethnically diverse than ever before. And these demographic changes have implications for the helping process. Culture shapes the meaning of body language, eye contact, and the role of the individual within the family unit. In addition, as helpers increase their awareness of and sensitivity to cultural differences, they must be especially cognizant of the differences not only between cultural groups, but among the members of one cultural group. For example, one cannot assume that all Puerto Ricans act or think alike or that all Asian Indians act or think alike. Helpers must continue to focus on the individual while continually being aware of the influence of ethnicity or culture.

The following introduction to Puerto Rican culture will provide you with general information that will help you understand Gloria, the client you will meet next, and the dilemma she faces. Without an understanding of her culture, you would miss critical information that allows you to be sensitive to what she thinks and how she acts. It will also give you a sense of the influence of culture upon the challenges she faces and the problems as she defines them.

UNDERSTANDING "HISPANIC"

Census 2000 in the United States used standards established by the Office of Management and Budget in 1997 to define the terms *Hispanic* or *Latino* as a person of Cuban, Mexican, Puerto Rican, South or Central American, or other Spanish culture or origin regardless of race (U.S. Census Bureau, 2001). Based on this definition, the U.S. Census Bureau reports that 43.2 million people in the United States are Hispanic or Latino (U.S. Census Bureau, 2006). It is estimated that some 2 million Puerto Ricans have migrated to the United States (Welcome to Puerto Rico, 2010) and are found in the metropolitan areas of every state, particularly in the northeastern United States. They probably refer to themselves as Puerto Ricans rather than as Americans although they consider themselves to be Americans. Their primary ethnicity is Hispanic; they use the term *Latino* to refer to peoples or countries using Romance languages, specifically in Latin America.

Migration from Puerto Rico to the United States is simple since no restrictions exist. In 1917, Puerto Ricans were made citizens of the United States and enjoy the rights of American citizens with the exception of voting in presidential and congressional elections. They pay no federal taxes. They may move to any part of the United States that they wish and have done so since the end of World War II when large-scale migration began. Today, many choose to migrate as contract labor hoping to improve their economic standing and eventually return to the island. Unfortunately, Puerto Ricans are overrepresented among the poor, have high unemployment, and often live in substandard housing (Sue & Sue, 2007). Although the literacy rate of Puerto Rico is 90 percent, instruction in school is Spanish; English is taught as part of the curriculum. This varied proficiency in English perhaps partly explains the lack of academic success for many Puerto Ricans in the United States. Migration of Puerto Ricans to the United States mainland, then, is not without problems.

The cultural and racial mix that represents Puerto Rico today began in the early 18th century when the Spaniards took Taino Indian women as brides and imported African slaves and Chinese men for labor. The arrival of Italians, French, Germans, and Lebanese followed in the 19th century. Most recently, Cuban immigrants arrived in great numbers during the 1960s. This historic intermingling of races both contributes to current racial harmony and to the physical appearances of the people that vary greatly.

RELIGION AND FAMILY

An appreciation of the role of religion and family in Puerto Rican culture is important in order to understand Puerto Ricans. Culture in Puerto Rico is organized around community life with the plaza at its center. The main building on the plaza is the church. Eighty-five percent of the population of Puerto Rico is Roman Catholic, thus the church plays a major role in the lives of the people. Religious beliefs that are integral to Puerto Rican life are: sacrifice is helpful to salvation, being charitable to others is desirable, and enduring wrongs against you is expected. The priest is a significant helping professional in the lives of the people. Help also comes from a belief in a folk system and folk medicine that explains and treats illness. Some Puerto Ricans believe that the spirit world can be contacted and prevailed upon to influence spirits through intermediaries. Many also regularly turn to folk medicine in the form of herbs, potions, and other remedies.

Religious practice also implies a pattern or network of intimate relationships, including related kinship and natural kinship, of which the family is central. Among Puerto Ricans living on the mainland United States, four family structures are significant. One is the extended family, which includes the natural kin and friends from the social network. This family structure is weakening as family members migrate permanently to the United States. Second, the nuclear family is becoming more common and includes the mother, father, and children. Third, the mixed family includes the nuclear family as well as children of another union or union of husband or wife. Finally, the single parent family is usually mother-based with children of one or more men, none of whom reside in the home. In Puerto Rican culture, divorce is less acceptable as a solution to marital difficulties than in the United States.

The family continues to be at the core of Puerto Rican culture. The family is valued over the individual; people gain prestige and status by demonstrating respect and cooperation in the family rather than individual achievement in the work force. While the network of family and friends offers unfailing support, the emotional involvement and obligations may also be a source of stress for the individual. Sex roles are clearly delineated with the father as the primary authority figure in the family. The traditional feminine role is to be submissive to the male, self-sacrificing, and restrained. For both males and females, role conflict is likely to occur if the male is unemployed, if the female is employed, or a combination of the two (Sue & Sue, 2007).

Those Puerto Ricans who migrate to the United States may experience a number of problems, many of them from external sources. If these individuals are poor, they may suffer from the stresses involved with inadequate food and housing, unemployment, and bureaucracies. The feelings of estrangement and displacement from the family, the island, and the culture may also cause difficulties. Language may present additional challenges with work and school. And finally, Puerto Ricans may encounter prejudice and discrimination in the larger community that may be beyond their control.

CASE STUDY: MEET GLORIA

LIST OF CHARACTERS

Gloria Martinez—Puerto Rican wife and mother of three who wishes to study in the United States

Mr. James—pastor of a church in Puerto Rico

Carlos Martinez—Gloria's husband who is disabled

Rosa—Gloria's youngest daughter who is 18

THE CASE Gloria Martinez is a 38-year-old Puerto Rican woman. She was born in Puerto Rico and spent her early years there. She lived for a time in the United States before returning to Puerto Rico where she resides now. At the time that she seeks help, she is married, has three children and two stepchildren, and has managed to obtain an education. She has an opportunity to study in the United States. As you will discover, she has spent many years taking care of others in her immediate and extended family. Herein lies her dilemma: if she pursues this move to further her education and to develop some valuable job skills, what will happen to her family?

The case study of Gloria is divided into two distinct helping events. The first helper is the pastor of a church in Puerto Rico. Gloria, unlike many Puerto Ricans and the rest of her family, is not Roman Catholic. Gloria is trying to decide if she should return to the United States to study. During their initial meeting, Mr. James has three goals. The first is to establish a relationship with Gloria, a member of the church he pastors. The second goal is problem identification. And the third goal for Mr. James is that he would like Gloria to leave their session feeling confident that they can work together to resolve the problem.

Mr. JAMES: Hello, Gloria. I'm glad to see you. I was pleased that you thought to call me and I've looked forward to talking with you. Did you have any problems finding my office?

GLORIA: No, I didn't. Your instructions were clear. I catch a ride with my brother.

Mr. JAMES: Good. Sometimes it's confusing because this is a big building. Now, what do you want to talk to me about?

GLORIA: You know I come to this church. I took sign language at the church. I want to work with deaf children. The class is over now and the teacher asked if I would like to study in the United States. I can return to Puerto Rico after I finish the program and work.

Mr. JAMES: Thinking about studying in the United States is very exciting for you—especially in an area that interests you.

GLORIA: Yes. I would really like to go back to the United States. My English is good and this would be a chance for me to get the training I need to work with the deaf. Puerto Rico desperately needs people who are trained in deaf education. I know I am smart enough to do this. I am the only one in my family who has finished high school and college.

This program lasts four months. It's an intensive program that trains people in sign language, deaf culture, and education of the deaf. It's exactly what I need and it's short. The students in the program are treated like university students, and they live in student apartments near the campus. There is even bus service, so I won't need a car. The church is willing to pay my tuition.

Mr. JAMES: You've investigated the program and you like what you've found out ... but it sounds like you have some reservations.

GLORIA: I don't know how I can leave my family. My mother and my uncles depend on me, and my husband and children need me, too. If I left, who would take care of my two daughters and my son? My husband's children don't need me so much. Ricardo, my husband's son, is in college in Puerto Rico and his girlfriend is in Iowa. He wants to go to the university in Iowa. We would be closer in the States than if I go to the U.S. and he stays in Puerto Rico. My husband's daughter, Consuela, is 19. Her boyfriend is in Puerto Rico, and I know she wants to be near him. I don't worry so much about her. She is grown and has her GED. She is studying to be a nurse's assistant. We had many problems with her because she didn't like to go to school. We were pleased when she decided to study nursing. As long as she studies something, it is fine with us. Her boyfriend is thinking about joining the Army, and I suspect they will get married. They are good kids. I raised them. They have education, and they've worked some. They'll be okay.

But my three—they still need me. Carlos, my husband, can't take care of them. He's disabled and takes medicine for his nerves. I wish I could take my family. The United States is a wonderful place for my kids to study and learn English. I would like for them to live in a different culture, but I don't know if they would even want to go. It would mean leaving our family who all live right here and their friends. And it would frighten them to think about going to a school where the language is one they don't know.

I know my mother and my uncles can't go. Their health is not good, and they are too old for such a trip, but I don't see how I can leave them. They depend on me to take them to the doctor, get their medicine, go to the grocery store, and everything. I don't know how I can leave them.

Mr. JAMES: You're concerned about how this will affect your family—and you wonder who will care for them if you go. Your family is very important to you. Tell me about them.

GLORIA: Yes, they are. My family is like most families in Puerto Rico. My mother lives next door to me, my brother lives next door to her, my other brother lives close by with his wife and his kids, my uncles live with my mother, because they don't have a home, and I live next to them. Everybody lives close together.

When I was in the fourth or fifth grade, my family moved to New York. Two of my brothers lived there and they sent for my father, who was disabled at that time because he had an accident. After my father was over there, then all of us followed him. There are five boys and five girls in my family. We have the same father and mother. My father also has a daughter who is about 53 or 54 now. She's my stepsister, but she was raised in New York since she was three years old by her aunt. Moving to New York was great for me. The language, the miniskirts, the music! It was very wild in New York! You didn't learn anything in school at that time. I had the feeling that we were passing grades just to pass.

Mr. JAMES: Sounds like living in New York was quite an experience for you.

GLORIA: Oh, yes. We lived in Brooklyn. My brothers and sisters still live in New York. They all live in the same building. And all my nieces and nephews, they get married and they moved to that building. There are two brothers and one sister in Puerto Rico, but they want to move to New York. When they move, they will live in one of my brothers' or sisters' apartments for awhile, until they get a job and get their own apartment.

Mr. JAMES: Did you stay in New York?

GLORIA: We moved back to Puerto Rico when I was in ninth grade. I ran away from home and went back to New York. I didn't like Puerto Rico, and so my friends helped me with the plane ticket and things like that. My brothers were waiting for me when I got to New York.

When I got to my friend's apartment building in a taxi, they were standing in front of the building. I was about 15 years old. They told me I had to live with them if I wanted to stay in New York, so I did. I went back to high school.

One day, I walked out of my brother's house, and they didn't see me again. I moved to New Jersey with a friend. She used to cook for the people who work on the farms—migrants. And I got a job doing migrant work. I picked strawberries, onions, stuff like that. They didn't request no ages or anything. One day my sister found out where I was, and she called me. She wanted to see me. When I went back to New York City, she told me how sick my parents were. She was going to get married and stay in New York, and she really wanted me to go back and take care of my mother and my father.

Mr. JAMES: And although you really liked New York, your family is very close and you felt you had to return.

GLORIA: Yes, I had to go back to Puerto Rico, but it was hard for me to live at home. Even though we are very close family, I used to have lots of problems with my mother and my father. I was the "black sheep" of the family. They used to say that. I was just different from everyone else at home. And I wanted many things, to do many things, and I was just too young and didn't have anyone to guide me.

Mr. JAMES: So your return to Puerto Rico was a difficult one—and the feeling of not fitting in was even stronger.

GLORIA: Yes. I am different from the rest of my family. In Puerto Rico, when I was young, girls were raised not even to finish high school if they didn't want to. They got married and had kids. So I ended up doing the same thing but not the way my parents wanted me to.

Mr. JAMES: Can you give me an example?

GLORIA: Well, I met Carlos at a party. We went out for a few months, and I lived with him instead of getting married. It was really hard for my parents. I was always doing the wrong thing for them. I felt like I was born in the wrong time and place. I should have been born now when it's more accepted. Six months later we did get married. He had a boy and a girl from his first marriage and we had three children, two girls and a boy.

Mr. JAMES: What was it like being married?

GLORIA: Carlos had a good job. He used to work with the telephone company. The reason my husband doesn't work now is because he is disabled from that job. He had an accident when I was pregnant with my last baby. That was one of the reasons that I decided to study and go to college. When I married him, I didn't know about paying bills. You see, I marry him, he pay for the house, he used to go shopping; anything I need, he used to take me, buy it, pay for it. I didn't know anything, even how much he earned. So when he had the accident and was in bed for a year, I just couldn't handle it. It was a terrible time. Five kids and I didn't know how to do anything. I didn't know where to pay this, where to pay that, where to send money for the house. I didn't know how to do anything. He was also dependent on me. I was taking care of him and five kids plus I needed to look after my mother.

Mr. JAMES: It must have been a hard time for you, knowing you were responsible for all those people but not knowing how you were going to survive this.

GLORIA: Yes, it was a very hard time for me. I was tired a lot and frustrated. At times I wondered if I was going to make it. Here I was taking care of all these people and I didn't know anything about money. And that's when I realized that I needed education. And I want my girls to be able to take care of themselves.

My husband, he is a good man. His first wife left him and the two children because she didn't want to be married anymore. In Puerto Rico, we marry young, before we know anything. His mother helped him with the children until I met him. He was a good worker and made good money. At least he always provided for us. Now he's disabled and may never work again. He was not a very good patient when he left the hospital. I had to wait on him a lot, and he got angry and frustrated because he couldn't do much for himself. It was a bad time for me. I was pregnant, had two small children plus his two, and I didn't know anything.

Mr. JAMES: Sounds like there were lots of demands on your time—and your energy.

GLORIA: After I had my last son, he was about two years old, I started watching TV. They had this program and they would give you this book in the library. I would watch the programs and study the books, and then I went to take classes for three months in the public school. I took my GED test and graduated. The next year I went to college, and that's what I've been doing all these years, working, studying, raising children.

Mr. JAMES: Studying and learning was important to you and you felt good about getting your GED and a college degree.

GLORIA: Yes, it was satisfying. And I worked too. I worked for an insurance company for a while doing secretarial work. It was okay. It didn't pay much but I was able to get out of the house for a while. With my husband's disability and his medical insurance, we were not so bad off. Of course, I still had to help my mother and my two uncles who live with her. I also worked part-time with the government in the Women, Infants, and Children Program, the WIC program. It was good experience. But I know now I want to work with the deaf here in Puerto Rico and I need this training. I don't know what I'm going to do.

It took Gloria a long time to decide to come to the United States to study. She wavered about staying in Puerto Rico or coming to the United States. She talked with her younger sister about their mother and uncles. The sister lives in Puerto Rico as do two of her brothers, but it was the sister who agreed to take care of them. Mr. James, her pastor, was encouraging. The program was only eight weeks, and he knew what her life was like. He recognized that she has spent most of her life taking care of family and children. This was a chance for Gloria to do something for herself that would provide her with the education and skills to work with the deaf. There are few people in Puerto Rico who have this training.

Once in the United States, Gloria began the training program. She received support from the faculty, fellow students, and the local Baptist church. Because she believed this was a good place for her children to go to school, to learn English, and to experience another culture, Gloria decided to remain for two more years to pursue a master's degree. Although there was much happiness at being reunited with her family, it was not long before problems occurred and Gloria, now a full-time student, sought help at the university counseling center.

COUNSELOR: I am glad that you have come to see me. Tell me about your life since you've been here at the university.

GLORIA: I really like my program and my classes. Everyone has been helpful, especially since my family is here now. My husband and my three younger kids arrived the end of October. We were all together and that was the most important thing to me.

COUNSELOR: You've missed your family a lot since you've been here.

GLORIA: Yes, I have. And I am so happy they are here. But none of them spoke English. Nothing.

COUNSELOR: That must have been tough for you.

GLORIA: Yes, it was. They needed me all the time. I enrolled the kids in school the week they arrived and their English is much better now. My husband, he does not speak English at all. He stays at the apartment all day because of his "nerves."

COUNSELOR: So your kids seem to be adjusting, but you're not sure about your husband.

GLORIA: That's right, although he will be okay. I am here to talk about some other problems I have. I don't know what to do about them.

COUNSELOR: Let's talk about them then.

GLORIA: In November, one of my daughters had a seizure. One night I heard a strange noise. I went into the bedroom of my youngest daughter who is 12 and I see that she was turning blue. So I called 911. I thought she was having a heart attack or something. An ambulance came and took her to the hospital. Well, it was all a fake. A false alarm. The doctor, he say that it was a reaction to the changes, the move from my country, my father, my mother, and leaving her friends. It was a tough move for her. She doesn't like changes. She is doing fine now and everything is okay. But it was an expensive fake. I'm still paying for it.

A week later, my kids were playing inside the apartment. They were playing, running after each other, and my oldest daughter was running after them. In Puerto Rico, my kids have lots of yard and patio to play. Here we have to stay inside because of the cold weather. I don't know how it happened but the door just locked on her fingers. Her fingers were just hanging. And that was the same week. I managed to put her inside my car. I bought a car that week. And I drive her to the hospital. The doctors have to do surgery on her fingers. It cost me $8,000. I owe right now $900 from that $8,000 because insurance that my children have from my country from my husband's company does not cover them here. So that's why I have to work so hard, sometimes two jobs. But her fingers are okay. The doctors sew them back, nerves and everything, to see if they survive and they did. This was in November.

COUNSELOR: Wondering how you are going to pay for all this is troubling you.

GLORIA: Yes, I am worried. I don't want to go to jail. And I'm worried about my family. In Puerto Rico the family is everything. My mother, my father, my uncles, my sister, my brothers are as important as my children. But here in the U.S. there is a different way of looking at it. My friend talked to me a lot. She'd say that sometimes you just have to decide. It's hard because my mother doesn't have many years to live, and I don't have many years to share with her.

I have many years to share with my children. I also think that I don't have the right to take my children's future away from them, because back home in Puerto Rico, there is nothing for them. There really isn't. So I have to make a very hard decision, weighing my mother against my children and who needs me the most. I know my mother needs me, too but I just cannot put my children's future in the background.

COUNSELOR: Adding to your concerns about money is feeling so torn about your responsibilities to your children and your mother in Puerto Rico. That must be really difficult for you.

GLORIA: Yes, it is. I feel guilty no matter how I think about it. On top of that, I am angry at my children. They can be 4.0 students, but because of boyfriends, friends, and playing, they are not really studying and bringing home the grades they need. It's not for me, it's for them. Sometimes I just sit back and I say "Is it worth it? Is it worth what I do?" I don't know. It's very confusing to think about.

COUNSELOR: Hmm. Tell me what's going on.

GLORIA: My kids are not the same as when they came here. They have changed so much. The culture has changed them a lot. For example, in my country, no matter how old you are, you have a lot of respect for what your parents say. You do what they tell you to do while you live at home. Once you get married, you still have respect for them, but you have your own life, too. While you are home, you respect everything your parents tell you. My oldest daughter, no matter how much I talk to her, she does not do what I tell her. She comes home late because she wants to be with her boyfriend all the time. I just feel like punching her sometimes. The other day I had a big talk with her and I told her: "This is it! You either follow the rule or I'm going to beat you up. While you live at home, you are still young. No matter if you're 20 years old, you are not old enough to do whatever you feel like doing."

COUNSELOR: The change in your children is very disturbing.

GLORIA: My other daughter talks back to me. In my country, kids don't do that. I mean you just put your head down and listen. For the first time, I gave her a big beating because of that. I hit her. I punched her and I slapped her and I hit her with my hands. It hurt me a lot but she straightened out. She doesn't answer me back anymore.

And my younger son used to stay home and study. Now all he wants to do is be outside playing. Staying in other people's house, friend's house. I am trying to give them values from Puerto Rico, but it's like those morals are not valid anymore for them.

Sex is a big problem. My daughter has friends her age having sex. She asked me the other day about how to avoid babies. I explain it to her. I tell her sex is a mistake, "If you do it, don't let me know it because I beat you." In Puerto Rico girls have to be virgins until they get married. And they better stay virgins until then. It's very hard here because my daughters see all the other girls having free sex.

COUNSELOR: You're concerned that your kids don't respect the values from Puerto Rico and you believe those are good values.

GLORIA: Yes and that's one of the reasons I want to move when I finish my degree. I am going to get more strict with them. I really am. I'm not going to give them the freedom they have here. I thought it was good for them to have a little bit of freedom going out with friends, staying over at friends' houses. I'm not going to permit that when we move and I've already told them.

COUNSELOR: Gloria, let me make sure I understand what's going on. Since your family arrived, you are facing a number of problems. One is about money and paying bills. A second has to do with what you think you should be doing for your family in Puerto Rico and for your family here. Finally, you have some serious concerns about the behavior of your children and the changes you see in them. Hmm. Which one would you like to tackle first?

The counselor and Gloria met for a second session. This session had a dual focus—making a plan to solve Gloria's economic problems and exploring issues related to Gloria's relationship with her children. The plan that focused on economic issues included outlining the debts, listing sources of income, planning repayment, and referring Gloria to other financial sources. Gloria felt relieved about the economic issues before she left the session. Focusing on her relationships with her children involved a very different approach. Gloria is very bright, and together she and the counselor examined the situation from her children's perspectives: the pressures and tasks that children are involved at different points of their life stages; the cross-cultural issues that both she and her kids were facing; and their possible feelings of not belonging in either world. While the problems did not disappear and cultural adjustments continued, Gloria's relationship with her children improved.

EPILOGUE

Gloria graduated with a master's degree in deaf education. Two months later, she moved her family to a southern city where the state school for the deaf is located. It also has a significant Hispanic population that is served by a Spanish newspaper and radio station. The presence of a Spanish-speaking population and culture has been beneficial to her husband. Because she now has a master's degree and is bilingual, finding a job was not difficult. While it has been a struggle to reach this point, Gloria continues to be excited and optimistic about the future.

CASE QUESTIONS

Gloria in Puerto Rico: Mr. James

1. How did Mr. James put Gloria at ease?

_____

_____

_____

_____

_____

_____

_____

_____

2. Did he accomplish the goals for the first meeting? Support your answer.

_____

_____

_____

_____

_____

_____

_____

_____

3. For what purposes are questions used in the interview?

_____

_____

_____

_____

_____

_____

_____

_____

4. How does Mr. James use communication skills to build a relationship with Gloria?

_____

_____

_____

_____

_____

_____

_____

5. What do you learn in the initial interview about Gloria's culture and its influence on her life?

_____

_____

_____

_____

_____

_____

_____

Gloria in the United States: The Counselor

6. Describe Gloria's life in the United States after her family's arrival.

_____

_____

_____

_____

_____

_____

_____

_____

7. How does the family adjust to living in the United States?

_____

_____

_____

_____

_____

_____

_____

8. How does the counselor encourage Gloria to describe her problems?

_____

_____

_____

_____

_____

_____

_____

9. Identify the stressors that Gloria experiences.

_____

_____

_____

_____

_____

_____

_____

10. What coping strategies does Gloria use to deal with her problems? Is she successful?

_____

_____

_____

_____

_____

_____

_____

_____

11. How does culture impact Gloria's life in the United States?

_____

_____

_____

_____

_____

_____

_____

EXERCISE: YOU AS THE HUMAN SERVICE PROFESSIONAL

Now that you have an understanding of some of the basic components of the helping process and are familiar with Gloria's case, answer the following questions:

1. Imagine that you are working with a Hispanic client. Discuss your biggest challenge.

_____

_____

_____

_____

_____

_____

2.   What are your impressions of Gloria as a client?

_____

_____

_____

_____

_____

_____

_____

3.   What strengths does she bring to the helping process? What challenges?

_____

_____

_____

_____

_____

_____

_____

4.   What would you do if your client told you she beat her daughter?

_____

_____

_____

_____

_____

_____

_____

5.   How would you help Gloria deal with the cultural conflicts she is experiencing?

_____

_____

_____

------

6. What qualities or characteristics do you have that would make you an effective crisis intervention worker?

ANOTHER PERSPECTIVE: LOIDA C. VELAQUEZ

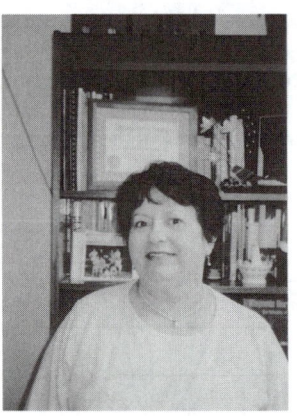

Loida C. Velaquez was born and raised in Puerto Rico. She moved to the continental United States with her husband and children. In 1979, she received a master's in educational psychology, and in 1993, a doctorate in technological and adult education.

Dr. Velaquez's entire professional life has been dedicated to working among minority groups. She has worked with the Department of Labor Job Corps program as director of training, and as a regional coordinator of a state protection and advocacy agency, a program responsible for the protection of the civil rights of people with disabilities. She is currently the administrator of a federally funded program for migrant and seasonal farm workers.

The marriage between anthropology, psychology, and sociology in human services is best reflected in this case. While some cultural groups are concerned with the self, Latino people are deeply engaged with their social and cultural contexts. This case can be better seen within a contextualist perspective where there is a weaving together of the individual and her social fabric. A contextualist perspective is characterized by an interest in understanding the diversity of patterns within the human experience as well as the realization of the heterogeneity within those patterns.

As a practitioner and as a Latina, I have incorporated this complexity into my professional and social life: I teach adult education graduate courses and I work in the administration of a program that helps students, mostly Latinos, to find in education a way to improve their lot in life. In the latest role, the program that I administer provides counseling; an educational curriculum geared toward achieving the GED; and assists the Latino students in the acculturation process to the dominant culture.

Like Gloria, I am also a Puerto Rican and have experienced firsthand the complexities of culture and identity: of being an American citizen and wanting to enjoy the advantages that residing in this country brings, of wanting to transform my identity while remaining true to my roots, of wanting to give to my children the best America has to offer but demanding from them a behavior that is rooted in the Hispanic values.

To better assist Gloria, we need to get a feeling for the contextual complexity of her perspective. Anthropologically she is a mixture of cultures: the Taino Indian that first inhabited Puerto Rico, the Spanish culture of the colonizers, the vestiges of the African culture of the slaves brought to the island to work in the sugar and coffee plantations. The psychological impact of colonization is something that has not been studied much and that mistakenly is often compared to the impacts of slavery. Added to that, is what Puerto Rican anthropologists have called *insularismo*, or the results of growing up in a very small island (100 miles long, 35 miles wide!), poor, rural, isolated, and tropical. She is in the United States of America but she is still thinking in insular terms.

Sociologically, she grew up with values, mores, and customs that are based on her Hispanic ethnicity. She admires the dominant culture of the United States, the opportunities it offers for education and professional development, even women's freedom; but she expects her children to develop as if they had never left Puerto Rico.

Psychologically, her identity is tied to her ethnicity and her culture. Although she has broken the stereotypical idea of the Latino woman who is expected to be submissive and quiet, she cannot accept her daughter developing an identity based on her own socializing culture. As soon as she can, she sends Rosa to Puerto Rico to stay with the grandmother, the same woman that Gloria defied many times and the home from which she ran away!

As her counselor, the first step I would take is to help Gloria realize that despite coming to counseling, she is a strong and resourceful woman. From a school dropout, a young bride, and mother from a rural and agriculturally based environment, she has developed into a professional and for all purposes the head of the family. She has coped with a disabled husband and left the support of the extended family to move her family to a southern town in [the] USA, to pursue a graduate degree and her dream of working with deaf children.

The second step would be to help her to understand how identity is culturally constructed and maybe assist her to develop an alternative self-conceptualization that is more fluid and adaptable. A self-concept that hopefully will assist her to negotiate in a better way the multiple roles she plays as a daughter, wife, mother, and provider.

EXERCISE: THE LAST WORD

You have the opportunity to have the last word on the concepts introduced and the case study presented. Based on what you have learned in this chapter, answer the following questions.

1. When you think about what you have read about the helping process, what stands out for you?

_____

_____

_____

_____

_____

_____

_____

_____

2. How did the chapter change your ideas and understanding about the helping process?

_____

_____

_____

_____

_____

_____

_____

_____

3. How will you use the information in this chapter in your own life and work?

_____

_____

_____

_____

_____

_____

_____

_____

4. What unanswered questions remain for you?

_____

_____

_____

_____

_____

_____

_____

_____

FOR FURTHER STUDY

BOOKS

Acosta-Belen, E., & Santiago, C. E. (2006). *Puerto Ricans in the United States: A contemporary portrait*. Boulder, CO: Lynne Rienner. This book represents a portrait of the Puerto Rican community today by reviewing Puerto Rico's colonial experience, the waves of migration, and commuter patterns.

Alvarez, J. (2010). *How the Garcia girls lost their accents*. Chapel Hill, NC: Algonquin Books. The story of four sisters who must adjust to life in the United States after fleeing from the Dominican Republic.

Arana, M. (2003). *American Chica: Two worlds, one childhood*. New York, NY: Delta. The author describes her years growing up in two cultures, that of Peru and the United States.

Day, F. (2003). *Latina and Latino voices in literature: Lives and works updated and expanded*. New York, NY: Greenwood. This is a source for young readers that includes author profiles, titles of works, and summaries of works. It is a good reference for teachers, librarians, and social service workers using contemporary literature to work with youth.

Davila, A. (2008). *Latino spin: Public image and the whitewashing of race*. New York, NY: NYU Press. The large and heterogeneous Latino population has been treated as both problem (immigrant) and opportunity (voters) by the spin often used to typecast the largest minority group in the United States. The author addresses popular images of Latinos and discusses the limitations of negative portrayals and attempts to address them.

MOVIES

The Motorcycle Diaries (2004). Director: Walter Salles Starring: Gael Garcia Bernal, Rodrigo De la Serna. *The Motorcycle Diaries* is based on the journals of Che Guevara, leader of the Cuban Revolution. In his memoirs, Guevara recounts adventures he, and best friend Alberto Granado, had while crossing South America by motorcycle in the early 1950s.

Selena (1997). Director: Gregory Nava. Starring: Jennifer Lopez, Jackie Guerra. The film portrays the life of Selena Quintanilla-Perez, a popular Latin singer, who died when she was 23. She began her singing career early and became the most popular Latin singer in the mid-1990s.

Under the Same Moon (2008). Director: Patricia Riggen Starring: Adrian Alonso. Kate del Castillo. This drama centers on a young boy's journey across the U.S./Mexican border to be reunited with his mother. The boy lives with his grandmother while his mother works as a maid in the United States, and hopes someday to send for her child. But when the grandmother dies unexpectedly, he must sneak across the border and seek out his mother.

WEB SITES

Explore the Web to learn more about the following:

Hispanic culture

National Hispanic Cultural Center

Welcome to Puerto Rico

Puerto Rico Resource Guide

Hispanic immigration

cross-culture counseling

Hispanic values

Latino counseling

Latino culture

Latino values

Puerto Rican counseling

Puerto Rican culture

Puerto Rican values

REFERENCES

U.S. Census Bureau. (2001). *The Hispanic population: Census 2000 brief*. Retrieved from http://www.census.gov/prod/2001pubs/c2kbr01-3pdf.

U.S. Census Bureau. (2006). *U.S. Hispanic population: 2006*. Retrieved from http://www.sensus.gove/population/socdemo/hispanic/cps2006/CPS_Powerpoint_2006.pdf.

Welcome to Puerto Rico. (2010). Retrieved from http://welcometopuertorico.org/people.htm.

Sue, D. W., & Sue, D. (2007). *Counseling the culturally diverse: Theory and practice*. New York, NY: John Wiley.

Working within a System

One way to describe the work of a human service professional is to consider the context or the environment in which it is delivered. This environment includes coworkers and supervisors, the agency or organization, and the wider social service sector, as well as the local, state, and national political, social, and economic climate. Agency environments define who receives what services, when they receive them, and how they receive these services. For those reasons, the environment is a critical component of understanding human services.

This chapter begins with an exercise that uses the content in Chapter 8 of *Introduction to Human Services, 7th ed.* to introduce the applications in this chapter. A second exercise requires you to write about the environment in which you have worked, are presently working, or volunteer. We review key ideas to help you better understand the environment and its influences. You will then have the opportunity to apply these concepts to your own work environment. Using the case study format, you will meet Steve Jackson, the director of Kirkpatrick Mental Health Center. His work and details of a particular crisis that he, his agency, and his community are facing with regard to community-based mental health will be presented. This case study provides you with an opportunity to better understand the importance of the environment of human service professionals as you respond to questions about Steve Jackson and the events of the crisis. Following your analysis, another perspective provides reactions to Steve Jackson and his case. Finally, you will have the "last word" as you reflect upon what you have learned in this chapter. Additional resources are listed for further exploration.

INTRODUCTION

Human service agencies and organizations that serve people are an important part of a community. Most communities have a local community services directory. Others may rely upon the yellow pages of a telephone directory or the Internet.

Using one of these resources where you currently live, answer the following questions:

1. Who publishes the resource you are using?

_____

_____

_____

_____

_____

2. How might you use an alphabetical index and a classified index or an Internet menu bar?

_____

_____

_____

_____

_____

3. What information does your resource provide about each agency, organization, or institution?

_____

_____

_____

_____

_____

4. Find an organization that provides direct help to people in need. Find an organization that provides membership opportunities for professionals.

_____

_____

_____

_____

5. Find a place to house and counsel a runaway adolescent. Name the place, location, telephone number, and describe how you found it.

_____

_____

_____

_____

_____

6. Find a place to get emergency food and clothing. Name the place, location, telephone number, and describe how you found it.

_____

_____

_____

_____

_____

7. Find three community services for elderly persons.

_____

_____

_____

_____

_____

8. Identify any available services for people who are blind.

_____

_____

_____

_____

_____

9. If you were unable to find any of these services, what would you do next?

_____

_____

_____

_____

_____

EXERCISE: WHAT ABOUT YOU?

Describe the environment in which you work or volunteer. Include the mission and goals of the business or agency. Describe the structure or chain of command of the management and employees. Discuss the work climate and culture, including whether it is positive or negative, friendly or unfriendly, and open or closed.

_____

_____

_____

_____

_____

KEY IDEAS

Effective helping includes assessing the environment in which human service professionals work. Successful helping occurs when environmental strengths support the helping process and environmental barriers become minimal influences.

MISSION

The mission or purpose of an agency or organization is communicated in a statement that is a summary of the guiding principles of the agency.

ORGANIZATIONAL STRUCTURE

The relationships among people and departments in an agency define its structure. Often, an organizational chart illustrates the lines of authority, information flow, and accountability by including boxes that represent offices, departments, and perhaps individuals.

FUNDING

The funding or financial support of an agency determines whether an agency is public or governmental, not-for-profit (voluntary), or for-profit. The distinction between public and not-for-profit agencies is not always clear because the not-for-profit agencies are increasingly providing services for public agencies on a contractual basis. The number of for-profit agencies is also increasing due to limited resources for voluntary agencies, reduced governmental spending, and changing political and economic times.

REVENUE

This term refers to the money an agency receives from four primary sources of funding: (1) federal, state, and local governments; (2) grants and contracts; (3) fees; and (4) donations. It is not unusual for agencies to receive money from multiple sources.

Organizational Climate

The conditions of the work environment that affect how people experience their work is the climate of the agency or organization. Based upon the values, attitudes, and feelings of people in the work setting, the climate influences how people perform their jobs and how they relate to clients.

Referral

Each professional helps a client by providing services, referring the client to other professionals when appropriate, or both. The professional assumes an important responsibility when referring a client. Assessing when to refer a client, determining to whom to refer, and making a successful referral are all components of this process. The reasons for referral vary from an inability to provide the service needed to a failure to help the client in question. Regardless of the reason for the referral, knowledge about other community resources and other helping professionals facilitate the process.

Promoting Change

The world of the human service delivery system is continually changing in response to political, economic, and social pressures. New client groups emerge, client needs alter, priorities shift, and methods of helping change. The dynamic nature of helping demands flexibility and willingness to change, and human service professionals view promoting change as an important role and responsibility. Questions at the foundation of the change process are:

What are client needs?

Does the change need to be agency or community based?

What are client roles in the process of change?

EXERCISE: YOU AND YOUR WORK ENVIRONMENT

This exercise focuses on you and the environment in which you work or volunteer. Before you begin to answer these questions, review the notes that you wrote for the previous exercise "What About You?" at the beginning of the chapter.

1. Does the mission of the place where you work or volunteer reflect what actually occurs there?

_____

_____

_____

_____

_____

_____

_____

_____

2. What aspects of your work or volunteer environment are you comfortable with?

_____

_____

_____

_____

_____

_____

_____

3. Which aspects would you like to change?

_____

_____

_____

_____

_____

_____

_____

_____

FOCUS: COMMUNITY MENTAL HEALTH

In the case study that follows, you will read about Steve Jackson, the director of a community mental health agency, who is challenged by providing services with limited resources to a population with expanding needs. Before we meet Steve and his colleagues, let's read about the history of community mental health in the United States and the challenges it faces today.

Much of the history of the treatment of the mentally ill in the United States reflects the history and development of state mental hospitals and represents the influences of welfare concerns. As early as 1824, Horace Mann advocated that care of the mentally ill should be the responsibility of the state since these individuals could not care for themselves. Others who made significant contributions to the care and treatment of the mentally ill were Dorothea Dix, a well-known reformer during the late 1800s, and Clifford Beers, a three-time mental patient in the early 20th century. During this time, the primary treatment remained institutionalization.

The concept of community-based mental health care for those with mental illness, emerged in the late 1950s, and received federal support when the Joint Commission on Mental Health and Illness recommended that no additional large state mental institutions be built. This was the impetus for deinstitutionalization of thousands of mentally ill patients from residential treatment. It was believed that many of these patients could function in communities with support. In 1963 that support came with the passage of the Community Mental Health Centers Act. Its goal was to establish a nationwide system of community mental health centers that would provide outpatient, community-based services (Gladding & Newsome, 2010; Woodside & McClam, 2012). This decision was the beginning of a national policy for mental health that expanded through the 1960s and 1970s.

During the 1970s many innovative programs developed to serve mentally ill clients. Innovations such as job-focused programs, family-centered services, halfway homes, and educational programs all offered new ways to support the mentally ill who were no longer institutionalized. The medically-prescribed use of psychotropic drugs helped stabilize clients, allowing them to increase their participation in mainstream society. Unfortunately, by the end of the 1970s, funding support from federal sources diminished, and many states were unable to increase their own contributions to mental health programs. Compounding the financial problem of providing community-based care to mentally ill people during the 1980s and 1990s were the growing pressures to fund health care, corrections, and welfare sectors. The lack of funding continues today even though the numbers of children, the homeless, substance abusers, and the elderly with mental health problems have risen dramatically.

Several criticisms of the current community mental health system explain some of the difficulties that community-based care has faced (Shore, 1992). First, those who promoted community mental health programs "overpromised" what could be done and who could be served. Since the federal funding was short-lived, there was never enough time or resources to integrate the mental health programs into community funding plans and priorities. Second, the number of individuals and families requiring services was underestimated and left professionals faced with an over demand for their services. This criticism in no way diminishes the efforts of the many professionals committed to serving mentally ill people on an outpatient basis. What these clients needed could not be provided with the resources available.

Politicians supported deinstitutionalization to save money, but these monies were never re-allocated to provide adequate services to the severely mentally ill who were discharged from hospitals. To live in the community, many individuals suffering from severe mental illness require intensive case management. Such services include working with clients weekly and often daily. Taking medications on a regular basis is a critical component of their treatment for it is the only chance these individuals have to function semi-independently. Professionals who provide effective intensive case management usually have no more than 8–10 clients. They provide support for vocational training, matching skills, capabilities, and education to employment, and assisting in activities of daily living such as washing clothes, bathing, cleaning house, managing money, accessing needed services, and many other responsibilities. For clients living with their families, the professional also often supports the family caregivers who assume these intensive case management responsibilities.

Many professionals ask if community mental health is a moot concept. Their question is based on the struggle through the years for adequate funding and for developing programs that truly meet the needs of the mentally ill and their families. The decline in funding at the federal, state, and local level presents challenges that must be addressed. Often those delivering community mental health services rely upon funding by providing services to those who can pay (either personally or have insurance); they also rely on them to finance those who cannot pay. Another strategy has been to increase caseloads in order to serve more clients, even though it may lower both the quality and intensity of services.

CASE STUDY: MEET STEVE JACKSON

LIST OF CHARACTERS

> **Steve Jackson**—director of the Kirkpatrick Mental Health Center
>
> **Simon**—mentally ill client who died in a hit-and-run accident
>
> **Pedro Ruiz**—mentally ill client who killed Luis Rey Ruiz
>
> **Ramon Ruiz**—Pedro's brother; Luis Rey Ruiz's father
>
> **Luis Rey Ruiz**—2-year-old son of Ramon Ruiz, killed by Pedro Ruiz
>
> **Ms. Thui**—board member
>
> **Dr. Bernstein**—professor of psychology, chairperson of the board
>
> **Mr. Seward**—bank president and board member
>
> **Ms. DeSelm**—member of both the KMHC board and the school board
>
> **Dr. Carol Weidimeier**—pediatrician and board member
>
> **Dr. Jime**—psychologist and board member
>
> **Ken Bonnett**—assistant executive director, friend of Steve Jackson
>
> **Louisa Jackson**—mother and confidant of Steve Jackson

The Case For the past two years, the staff of Kirkpatrick Mental Health Center (KMHC), under the leadership of Steve Jackson, has reorganized and retrained in an attempt to address service demands. Two recent deaths in the community have served as a catalyst for the staff to bring attention to the plight of the clients and the dilemma of the agency. In response to the staff request, Steve Jackson speaks to his board of directors, challenging them to address the issues within the broader community.

Steve Jackson slowly walked into the office on Monday morning. He was still thinking about the staff meeting held in his office last Friday and the ensuing events of the weekend. The weekly meeting of the Kirkpatrick Mental Health Center staff had been a disaster, despite his best efforts. But from the Monday morning perspective, he could have expected it. The staff had been working under tremendous pressure for the past six years, and the last two years had been particularly difficult. And the last six months—well, it seemed that everything was going downhill.

For the staff, the problems were endless, and at a quick glance, an easy answer was that deinstitutionalization of the mentally ill was simply not working. In reality, that explanation was too simple. From the client perspective, there were too few services available, many of which were inaccessible. Clients, their families, and the mental health staff did not receive consistent support. Even basics such as food, housing, and medical care were of low quality. Basically, the clients had nowhere to go for the services they needed.

For several years the clients were the ones who really suffered, and now the staff was also troubled. They saw failure every day with little hope of helping many of their clients. For the past 15 years, the number of those housed in the state mental institution had decreased. The institutional census had dropped from 2,819 to 154. Since most of the clients were no longer being housed in the local state mental institution, they needed alternative housing. Some ended up with family or friends who did not want the heavy responsibility of their care. Some chronic clients were illtreated at home or ended up dismissed by frustrated families who could not devote their lives to these mentally ill individuals. Clients sought shelter in mission homes, on the streets, and in the jails. Sometimes they were lucky enough to find lodges, single-room dwellings, or halfway houses, but many were not allowed to remain in these places because of deviant behavior or lack of money. In fact, some even checked back into the mental institution for a brief stay when they could find no other source of housing and could convince officials that they were dangerous to themselves or to others. Some patients had been admitted and discharged from 10 to 40 times in the past few years, creating a "revolving door" syndrome.

Two deaths within a month of each other finally brought the crisis to a head with the staff at the Kirkpatrick Mental Health Center. Last month, a patient named Simon, whom they had first served ten years ago at the beginning of his deinstitutionalization, was a victim of vehicular homicide. He was on the streets in a quiet part of town late Thursday evening. As he was crossing the street in the middle of a block, he was hit by a car. He died just before midnight from injuries he sustained in the hit-and-run accident. Information about the death circulated to board members and staff on the internal Internet communication system and text message board. Almost everyone knew about the death Friday morning before work. Tragic deaths had come before to the agency's clients, but Simon's death was felt especially hard by the staff.

Two years ago, the agency had decided to use him as a test case to challenge the "least restrictive environment" principle used to determine the appropriate therapeutic setting for the chronically mentally ill client. The state mental hospital said that Simon did not need long-term institutionalization to receive the treatment he needed and discharged him. As they were responsible for Simon's follow-up care, the agency decided to give Simon the best treatment they could offer, making careful notes on his progress.

The mental health center staff worked with Simon, but they had never felt hopeful that he could exist in a deinstitutionalized environment. The "revolving door" had been an integral part of his treatment from the beginning. Case managers would struggle to support his family, administer his medication, teach him basic living skills, and assist with his transition to day programs and group homes. Simon could somewhat function while on medication, but after a time, he would forget to take it. Once he was off the medication, his disruptive behavior made him an unattractive member of any group whether it be a family, day group, or group home. Ironically, the agency had requested Simon's readmission to the state hospital the day of his death. They asked for a special hearing of his treatment team, hoping to review his ten-year history with the hospital staff. This review was never held because of Simon's untimely death.

Summary Points for Simon

- Deinstitutionalized ten years ago
- Revolving door: in and out of state hospital last two years
- Two years ago used as test case for "least restrictive environment"
- Day of death, agency requests Simon's readmission to the state hospital
- Simon was victim of vehicular homicide

The second death, the murder of Luis Rey, occurred last Tuesday. Again the KMHC board and the staff were immediately informed. Staff discussed the death at last Friday's meeting about the crisis. Luis Rey was the 2-year-old son of Ramon Ruiz. Ramon's brother, Pedro, had been a client with the agency for the past four years. He suffered from paranoid schizophrenia, and he had been institutionalized eight times in the past year. His brother wanted to care for him and opposed institutionalization.

The agency had worked with the family, but had not always been able to give them what they needed. They were unable to find support services as the major problems were the lack of money and transportation. Pedro lived a good distance from the bus line and could not find a way to get to the outpatient clinic or to the recreational center. He also had too much money to qualify for Medicaid and not enough money to pay for the services he needed. Pedro demonstrated violent tendencies and needed to be medicated at all times. At home, Pedro's refusal of medication initiated a cycle common for him and many chronically mentally ill. He moved from the institution to home because his behavior stabilized with medication, and he was no longer dangerous to himself or others. Once removed from supervision, he refused or forgot to take his medication. Then, slowly, the old symptoms returned until his behavior warranted readmission to the hospital.

Summary Points for Pedro Ruiz

- Pedro has been a client with the agency for four years
- Institutionalized eight times during the past year
- Needs continuing medication to soothe violent behavior
- Consistently on/off medication
- Kills his nephew, Luis Rey, while off medication

After his most recent release from the hospital, Pedro refused to take his medication on the first day back in Ramon's home. Five nights later, he could not sleep and spent the night using scissors to bang on the pans in the kitchen and cut up the curtains. Early the next morning, he used the same scissors to stab his nephew, Luis Rey, to death. His father, Ramon found the boy dead in his bed, called the police, and then sat with his brother, Pedro on the front steps as they waited for the unmarked car. Ramon stayed behind on the steps grieving for his family and waiting for the ambulance to take the body of his baby boy to the morgue.

The staff was very affected by this death and met Tuesday evening to discuss the failure of the agency and the community to protect the life of Luis Rey. Many of the staff members were angry and determined that this incident should not go unnoticed. They felt it should be an impetus for major change. The strong emotions vented in this meeting were preceded by similar Internet exchanges. By the end of the meeting, the staff had agreed to ask for three things: as individuals they needed to advocate for the treatment of their clients; the agency needed to assume responsibility for advocacy in the community; and the community as a whole needed to address the problem of the mentally ill. Their first step in accomplishing these goals would be to convince their director, Steve Jackson that a radical approach was needed. Several staff members met Wednesday night to plan their strategy for Friday's meeting.

From the staff's perspective, the Friday meeting was even more successful than they could have hoped. Their rage and their vehemence shook Steve, but he listened carefully to all they had to say. His reasonableness had calmed their anger, but they did not want to lose their emotion. At the conclusion of the meeting, the staff demanded action and attention to their three demands. Steve promised that he would carefully consider their concerns and meet with them next week.

THE DIRECTOR'S PERSPECTIVE   *From Steve Jackson's perspective, Friday's staff meeting did not begin well. He had prepared an agenda and began the meeting by speaking of the death of Luis Rey. His comments initiated a discussion that supplanted the original agenda. The staff had come to the meeting partially organized, and they intended to focus the staff meeting on the whole problem, not just on individual patients.*

What the staff did not know was that Steve was in complete agreement with their demands. He knew about the crisis in community mental health, but he felt his responsibility was to focus on the services provided by his agency. What had been disconcerting for him were his feelings of hopelessness and despair over the last year. It seemed that no matter what steps he took at the agency, the final result was failure. The agency could not meet the needs of the clients it served. Steve knew now that he had to share this revelation with his board of directors. His two tasks in communicating with them were to convince them of the impossible situation facing the agency and the necessity of facing the dilemma with a community effort. To that end, he called an emergency meeting of his board of directors for Sunday afternoon. Steve spent all day Saturday preparing for the Sunday meeting, knowing that he had to get their attention.

THE BOARD MEETING   *Sunday was a difficult day for Steve. He woke up early, unable to sleep because of the anticipated afternoon meeting. He prepared and fine-tuned his presentation several times. He reviewed the sequence of events that had brought him to this day (see Table 8.1).*

TABLE 8.1	SEQUENCE OF EVENTS
One month ago	Simon's death
Tuesday morning	Murder of Luis Rey
Tuesday evening	Staff meets
Wednesday evening	Staff meets again
Friday	Staff meeting with Steve Jackson
Sunday afternoon	Board of directors of Kirkpatrick Mental Health Center meet with Steve Jackson

A walk, attendance at church, and lunch with his family did nothing to distract Steve from his upcoming meeting at 2:00 P.M. He knew that it just had to go right. By 1:30 P.M., he was in the conference room with his computer turned on and connected to the projector. He had practiced the presentation twice; he could not afford for anything to go wrong. The members of the board of the Kirkpatrick Mental Health Center mostly came in one at a time as they always did. Ms. Thui arrived first. Always cheerful, she made her greetings and asked how long the meeting would last. Her daughter was performing in a string quartet later that day at 4:00 P.M. Dr. Bernstein, a professor of psychology from the university and chairperson of the board, arrived next. He brought papers just in case the meeting started late. He graded final exams and seemed preoccupied with end of the term concerns. Then came Mr. Seward, president of a local bank, Ms. DeSelm, a member of the school board, and Dr. Carol Weidimeier, a pediatrician and the newest member of the board. She brought regrets from Dr. Jime, a psychologist in private practice, who was at home with the flu.

Steve had decided to start quietly with his presentation, hoping to keep the board's interest and pique their curiosity about the nature of the emergency. He had plenty of information with which to grab their attention, but he wanted them to understand the history of the problem. So he related a short history of community mental health, a concept that embodied the principles of social reform in the post-World War II years. He explained that in 1955 over 560,000 patients were institutionalized for mental disorders in the United States, and now, after deinstitutionalization, approximately 140,000 patients were institutionalized. This was a reduction nationwide of over 70 percent. Steve then described the two main thrusts in the deinstitutionalization movement: a shift in the population from the institution to the community and with fewer admissions, treatment for newly diagnosed individuals would be found now in that community.

Steve looked at his audience. During his summary of the history of deinstitutionalization, he had not lost center stage. But he could feel Mr. Seward and Dr. Weidimeier were beginning to wonder when he would present the major point. His next PowerPoint slide placed the discussion in the center of the board's interest, their own agency.

"Let's look at the agency in 1969 when it first opened its doors," Steve continued. "One of you served on that first board and three of you lived in this city at the time. Let's look at Kirkpatrick Mental Health Center in 1969. The major goal of this center was to meet the mental health needs of this community. This goal

included providing services for the chronically mentally ill, deinstitutionalized mentally ill, those needing crisis or emergency care, and anyone in the community in need of preventative services. The services we offered were outpatient services, 24-hour emergency service, consultation, and education. We had ten staff on the community team, as we called it then: one full-time administrator, one half-time administrator, one half-time psychiatrist, two therapists, two aides, three case managers, and a driver. That first year we provided intake for over 500 clients. These included clients from the community and those who were entering the community from the institution for the first time. We served 70 in a day treatment program; 90 in individual therapy; we helped 200 in their transition to the community; we referred 100 to other agencies."

Looking over the top of his computer, Steve could watch his audience closely. He saw glimmers of interest while the board members each thought about those early days from their own perspectives. Mr. Seward was on that first board, and he served for five years. He reflected those were both exciting and tough times for the agency. At that time, Mr. Kruster was the director, and he was exactly the right choice. His two greatest skills were setting goals and motivating people. Seward laughed to himself as he thought about Kruster who thought the center would save the world and eradicate mental illness. He then turned his attention back to Steve Jackson, thinking how times have changed.

Carol Weidimeier felt burdened by this meeting and hearing the brief history only increased her despair. She had agreed to be on this board because she wanted to make a difference in the mental health community. According to the history, as told by Steve Jackson, someone had forgotten to ask some basic questions when they planned this new system of service delivery. Steve, speaking in a lower voice than usual, broke into her thoughts. He raised his voice as he started to contrast the past with today, introducing a new graphic on the screen with the left column open and the right column covered.

The board saw immediately the changes over the last 30 years. Steve then reviewed the current status of the organization. "The goals of this agency have not changed much from the goals that were established in 1969. We are still committed to meeting the mental health needs of the community, providing direct treatment and preventive efforts. The client population we serve also remains the same. But we have expanded our services to meet the diverse needs of our clients. The original services are still offered, but we have added special services to family, independent living coaching, and liaison for housing. We have new programs to serve the homeless and our numbers of mentally ill elderly are increasing. These additions were in direct response to the needs of our clients. Today, we have a staff of over 50 professionals administering and providing mental health services. Last year, we conducted initial interviews with over 2,000 clients. We served over 1,000 of those clients in one or more of our programs, and we referred over 500 to other agencies."

The pace of his presentation and his voice took on a hurried effect as Steve wanted his listeners to feel his urgency; the information about the current situation was not to be the highlight of this presentation. The final category on the right column of this graphic was titled "On Hold." Otherwise, the screen was blank. Steve had chosen this title carefully to reflect the crisis that was occurring in the community in mental health care today. He wanted the board to feel the hopelessness that his staff felt and also to convey the sense of possibilities that he was going to propose. He then told his audience about the seriousness of the next piece of information they were to receive; it concerned the future. He brought up the next screen so everyone in the room could focus on the current problems. Steve now slowed down and let the information speak for its self. He asked now that none speak until he was finished; but he passed out sheets of paper so the board could jot down their questions as they listened. He then reviewed the overhead.

1. **Intake.** *The agency is already scheduled six months ahead. This includes referrals from the state mental institution, the Department of Corrections, Child and Family Services, private practice physicians and psychiatrists, ministers, local nursing homes, the Department of Health, homeless shelters, elder protective services, and others. The six months of scheduling represented over 1,500 clients and their families; Steve reminded the board that intake was only the first step and did not represent any treatment.*

2. **Service demand.** *In the last month, the intake services had received calls from more than 275 individuals or professionals, or approximately nine calls a day, wanting services but not able to wait the six months for an appointment.*

3. **Emergency services.** *More than 50 people a week are seen in the time slots reserved for emergencies. Each week another 50 are turned down because there are no services available.*

4. **Case management.** *The caseload of each manager is 150. This number means that they have little time for individual management and follow-through with these clients. Deinstitutionalization, as a concept, was intended to be flexible and easy to alter depending upon the needs of the mentally ill it served.*

5. **Referrals.** *The agency makes referrals to other agencies for needed services. During the last six months, incomplete referrals numbered over 680. Not only can the agency not meet the need, other agencies are also feeling the same pressure.*

6. **Shortage of services in the community.** *There are more than 3,000 chronically mentally ill in this community, with needs for housing, vocational rehabilitation, medication, and social interaction. Some need specialized services if they are dually diagnosed as substance abusers as well. There is housing in the community for 1,250, vocational rehabilitation for 870, proactive medical availability for 1,300, and places that provide social support for approximately 590.*

Steve looked up and continued. "These past two years this agency has been involved in a commitment to provide more quality services. We have reorganized twice to meet the following goals: to better serve the clients; to serve more clients; and to provide better staff support. In the last six months, the innovations have included staff working in pairs to serve more clients in groups; more in-service for staff; using up-to-date treatment techniques; and team meetings with members of other agencies to problem-solve and improve communication. We finally realize the problem is bigger than this agency or our individual efforts."

Steve now lowered his head. He would need his strength to deliver this final request, and he decided to take the formal approach. "Members of the board, I think that you can see from this presentation that we are facing a grave situation *in mental health in this agency and in our community. We are in danger of not meeting all our goals and objectives, trading them for just surviving and hanging on. I would like to propose that we provide a leadership role within the community to solve this problem. The reason that I ask for your support and your leadership is that this is a very difficult task. As you know, our community is not usually a community in common. And in a time of scarce resources the isolation and distrust is even more than usual. Although individual staff members work together, we need a vision of cooperation that begins at the top. And we need the wisdom to ask all involved administrators, staff, and consumers to help us address this problem communitywide. If we assume a leadership role, it will cost us in time and money and political problems. But I am afraid if we do not assume this responsibility, then the picture of mental health in our community will continue to worsen. I now invite you to share your ideas about this proposal."*

At the Sunday emergency meeting of the board of directors, all agreed that the impassioned pleas from Steve deserved more thought and discussion. The decision to do something beyond the agency focus was placed on the agenda of the next regular monthly meeting, which was scheduled for the following Friday afternoon. Each board member committed to bringing some considerations about the matter. All were in accord that the issue was too important for them to act too quickly, but several cautioned that they could also talk the issue to death.

Steve met with his staff early on Monday morning to report the results of the Sunday board meeting. He urged them to be patient and also encouraged them to develop several strategies that could be distributed to the board members to be considered during the decision-making process. Steve planned to have lunch that week with several of his counterparts in other mental health agencies and discuss the issues. Whatever goals and strategies developed, he believed that cooperation in the community was the key.

On Tuesday Steve met with Ken Bonnett, a trusted colleague for more than ten years, who was assistant executive director at the local state mental institution. In his conversation with Ken, he shared the events of the past week. He discussed with Ken what he thought were the needs of the chronically mentally ill. He also challenged him to think of the last time the community banded together to work on mental health issues. Unfortunately, Ken could not think of even one occasion. But he did tell Steve the story of the media's assault on the mental hospital in the mid-1960s. It was a nightmare that Steve did not want to repeat. Ken cautioned that unfavorable press without positive outcomes would leave mental health services in worse straits than before this most recent attempt to improve the situation.

On Wednesday at 7:00 P.M., after an hour of paperwork in a quiet office, Steve joined his mother for supper. Although in her 70s, Louisa Jackson still maintained an interest in civic affairs, and her son had respect for her opinions. She was well-schooled in promoting change and had been a community organizer even before that phrase had become popular. When he was just a small boy entering school, his mother worked in the janitor's broom closet, teaching special reading classes to children who could not read. The story he heard from his mother's friends was that she bullied the principal into letting her have the space and the students in return for her support at local parent meetings. Her advice was to start small and gain

TABLE **8.2** | SEQUENCE OF EVENTS

Monday morning	Staff meeting
	Staff develops questionnaire
Tuesday	Jackson meets with Ken Bonnett
Wednesday	Staff meeting
	Board gathers information
Friday	Board meeting—appointment of task force
5 weeks later	Development of "white paper"
6 weeks later	Task force members meet with board members
7 weeks later	Special board meeting—task force presents white paper
Last Thursday in July	Task force meets with Ministerial Alliance members
First Tuesday in August	Task force meets with Mental Health Association board

support at the grass roots level. She cautioned against only involving "big time administrators."

Steve was not the only person who focused on the dilemma presented at the Sunday board meeting. (See Table 8.2.) The staff of Kirkpatrick held three meetings during the week in an effort to get the input of every staff member. They had decided to talk face-to-face. On Monday, several of the staff developed a questionnaire that would help them determine what everyone believed were the problems and what they would propose. They kept the questionnaire simple, putting an emphasis on having input from all of the staff. They were not able to get 100 percent cooperation, but they did manage to collect surveys from more than 45 staff members. The results of the survey illustrated the wide diversity of opinions within the staff. But three conclusions stood out: over 80 percent thought some action should be taken by the community to address the mental health problems; almost 70 percent of the respondents were willing to participate in the change process; but some 62 percent of the staff were pessimistic that change could be effected.

Many members of the board were also preoccupied during the week with this challenge. Three of them spent time on the telephone talking to their friends and colleagues and others in the mental health field. Carol Weidimeier, the pediatrician, decided to collect information about her patients and she called three other colleagues to assemble similar data. She asked them how many patients they had, the percentage who need mental health services (by their own diagnosis), the percentage who report receiving mental health services, the percentage they have referred for mental health services, and the results of the referrals. It was a short turnaround time for this type of information, but Carol was able to complete her statistics and two of the three other pediatricians sent theirs to her by Friday morning.

Ms. DeSelm had been on two other human service boards during the past 20 years, and she had met many people in the mental health arena. She called two of them to ask about their experiences with the mental health needs in the area. She then had lunch with the two members of the board of the local Mental Health Association to assess their reactions to a communitywide focus. As she expected, she received diverse opinions. The discussion had been a good one with much dialogue on the political dimensions of the problem. The best outcome was a promise from them that they would support their agency's discussion of a joint project.

THE FRIDAY BOARD MEETING *The Friday board meeting began on time. Each of the board members was there early and Dr. Jime, just back from his illness, sat at the table looking expectantly at his fellow members. He had missed the meeting on Sunday, but had heard about it from four other members. He was glad to be back in order to participate in this important meeting. Steve took his place at the table, and the chair, Dr. Bernstein, began the meeting. First, he introduced several items of business that, because of time pressures, had to be taken care of at this meeting. He then placed in committee several issues that needed study and future resolution. Everyone held their breath as he introduced the next item of business: planning for provision of mental health services for the community. He knew that each person around the table had important things to say and, even more importantly, they wanted to be heard. To that end, Bernstein decided to record the information presented on big flipcharts around the room. When each was finished, the information would be visible for everyone to see. Dr. Jime agreed to take notes on the flipcharts. The order of each speaker was determined by the seating arrangement and the chair called on Ms. Thui first. Everyone presented their information and the ideas they had gathered since Sunday. There was overwhelming support to begin to address the needs of both the client population and the professionals committed to working with them.*

The conclusion of the meeting was to appoint a task force to work together to plan a strategy to improve the delivery of mental health in the community. There would be five members on this community task force: a board and staff member from the Kirkpatrick Mental Health Center, a board and staff member from the staff of the Mental Health Association, and a member of the local Ministerial Alliance. The task force was to meet and report back to the next regular board meeting next month. The board meeting was then adjourned.

Several left the meeting wishing that things could move a little faster. Others left feeling that the agency had taken on too much. Still others felt that the issues of the agency had been pushed aside, and they did not want the board to lose sight of the purpose of the board, to assist in the running of the agency. All of the members were sure, however, that this issue did require their attention.

CASE QUESTIONS

    1. Describe the staff mentioned in this case study.

_____

_____

_____

_____

_____

_____

_____

_____

2. Construct an organizational chart that includes board members. Assign names when you know them.

_____

_____

_____

_____

_____

_____

_____

3. Write a mission statement for Kirkpatrick Mental Health Center.

_____

_____

_____

_____

_____

_____

_____

4. Describe the working environment at Kirkpatrick Mental Health Center.

_____

_____

_____

_____

_____

_____

_____

5. The board and staff are coping with change. Describe one incident of change in the case study.

_____

_____

_____

_____

_____

_____

_____

_____

6. At Kirkpatrick Mental Health Center, what part does referral play in meeting client needs?

_____

_____

_____

_____

_____

_____

_____

7. Why is Steve Jackson promoting change in community-based mental health care?

_____

_____

_____

_____

_____

_____

_____

8. What do you think will happen to KMHC?

_____

_____

_____

_____

_____

_____

_____

_____

EXERCISE: YOU AS THE HUMAN SERVICE PROFESSIONAL

Now that you have an understanding of the importance of the environment of an agency, answer the following questions:

1. What is your reaction to this case?

_____

_____

_____

_____

_____

_____

_____

_____

2. What are the challenges working with the chronically mentally ill?

_____

_____

_____

_____

_____

_____

3. How do you feel about the two deaths in the case study?

_____

_____

_____

_____

_____

_____

4. Assume that you are a colleague of Steve Jackson's. Think about the advice you would give him about his particular crisis at KMHC.

_____

_____

_____

_____

_____

_____

_____

_____

5. How would you describe Steve Jackson's leadership at KMHC?

_____

_____

_____

_____

_____

_____

_____

_____

ANOTHER PERSPECTIVE: MARCIA KATZ

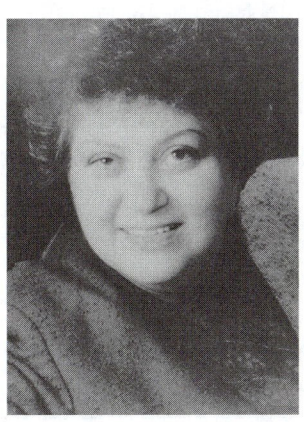

As a board member at a community mental health center, Marcia Katz offers her perspective of Kirkpatrick Mental Health Center. Dr. Katz has a Ph.D. in nuclear engineering and has held positions as a tenured associate professor, a visiting lecturer in Brazil, a researcher in France, and as a White House Fellow. She has received numerous teaching and research awards, and has served as a board member in a number of other organizations, including the local Association of Women Executives and her synagogue and the Jewish Federation.

As I read "Focus: Community Mental Health," I relived my experience on the board of a community mental health center, a not-for-profit, community-based, nongovernmental agency, established by concerned citizens more than 50 years ago. Over the course of three terms, I served on the board's executive, financial, and personnel committees, and chaired the committee that produced the annual report.

At first, the center was active in only one urban county. Over the years the scope increased in both services delivered and areas served, necessitated by the changes in needs and in funding sources for mental health services. It grew in a planned, orderly manner under inventive leadership—both financial and medical. When it became evident that additional funding was necessary, another independent, not-for-profit entity was established to raise [the funding].

Staff worked under tremendous pressures as in the depicted Kirkpatrick Mental Health Center, but there was never a morale problem. The director and the other administrators worked at heading off problems and the staff and board members were consulted for solution ideas.

The Kirkpatrick case study is realistic. Steve Jackson and the board of the Kirkpatrick Mental Health Center faced the problems similar to the real-life situations I saw. In the scenario, client transportation presented a difficulty. Transportation was such an essential part of treatment and as such was always part of our clients' treatment plans. One of our clients died in circumstances reminiscent of the tragic death of Luis Ruiz.

In contrast to the agency depicted, my experience was with a center whose leadership was "on top of" changes in mental health delivery system and kept the board "in the know" also. The member's education began each year with extensive orientation sessions and continued at each of the monthly meetings with meaty, technical reports by the frontline staff members. Board members were invited to the staff's professional in-service training sessions where I learned a lot about treatment of the mentally ill; for example, evidence of a client's improving mental health is a widening circle of friends, so the recreational drop-in center is essential and there is a new medication that works miracles for schizophrenic clients and does not have detrimental side effects.

My service on the board was educational, fulfilling, and challenging. I was able to contribute from my seemingly unrelated background because of the professional abilities of the president and other administrative staff. My years of service would not have been as gratifying without it.

EXERCISE: THE LAST WORD

You have the opportunity to have the last word on the terms introduced and the case study presented. Based on what you have learned in this chapter, answer the following questions:

1. When you think about what you have learned about the environment and human services, what stands out for you?

_____

_____

_____

_____

_____

_____

_____

_____

2. How did the chapter change your ideas and understanding about the influence of the environment on human services?

_____

_____

_____

_____

_____

_____

_____

3. How will you use the information in this chapter in your own life and work?

_____

_____

_____

_____

_____

_____

_____

4. What questions remain unanswered for you?

_____

_____

_____

_____

_____

_____

FOR FURTHER STUDY

Books

Bhugra, D. (Ed.) (2007). *Homelessness and mental health*. Cambridge, UK: Cambridge University Press. As a global perspective on homelessness, this book brings together the experiences of mental health teams from around the world in addressing the problems of mental illness in the homeless.

Gladding, S. T., & Newsome, D. W. (2010). *Clinical mental health counseling in community and agency settings*. Upper Saddle River, NJ: Prentice Hall. This book covers all aspects of community counseling, including roles, functions, settings, and client populations.

Lamb, R. H., & Weinberger, L. E. (Eds.). (2001). *Deinstitutionalization: Promise and problems: New directions for mental health services #90*. San Francisco, CA: Jossey-Bass. An examination of the positive and negative effects of deinstitutionalization is the focus of this book. Issues addressed include the use of community alternatives to state hospitalization; the large numbers of mentally ill persons who have found their way into the criminal justice system; the community treatment of mentally ill offenders; and psychiatric rehabilitation.

Roberts, A. R. (Ed.). (2000). *Crisis intervention handbook: Assessment, treatment, and research*. Oxford, UK: Oxford University Press. Timely and comprehensive help for crisis intervention teams is available in this handbook, which prepares the crisis counselor for rapid assessment and intervention in the 21st century. It focuses on crisis intervention services for persons who are victims of natural disasters, school-based and home-based violence, violent crimes, and personal or family crises.

Torrey, E. F. (2008). *The insanity offense: How America's failure to treat the seriously mentally ill endangers its citizens*. New York, NY: W.W. Norton. The author's thesis is that deinstitutionalizing mental patients, closing mental hospitals and turning schizophrenics and manic-depressives out onto the streets has contributed to an increasing number of violent attacks, murders, and suicides.

Movies

As Good As It Gets (1997). Director: James L. Brooks. Starring: Jack Nicholson, Helen Hunt, Greg Kinnear. Jack Nicholson plays a bigoted, obsessive-compulsive writer who finds his life turned upside down when neighboring gay artist (Kinnear) is brutally beaten and, when hospitalized, entrusts the care of his dog to Melvin (Nicholson). In addition, Carol (Hunt), the only waitress who will tolerate him, leaves work to care for her sick son, making it impossible for Melvin to have breakfast.

Girl, Interrupted (1999). Director: James Mangold. Starring: Winona Ryder, Angelina Jolie. Based on writer Susanna Kaysen's account of her 18-month stay in a mental hospital in the 1960s, this movie depicts life in a private mental hospital. Patients include a pathological liar, a sociopath, a sexually abused young woman, and a burn victim. Issues include confidentiality, patient compliance, staff roles and responsibilities, and institutionalization.

Monk. Starring: Tony Shalhoub, Stanley Kamel. *Monk* is a television series about Adrian Monk, a former San Francisco Police Department star, who developed an extreme case of obsessive-compulsive disorder after the still unsolved murder of his wife. Now a private consultant, Monk has supportive friends and a gifted therapist who help him cope with his phobias and obsessions.

The Soloist. (2009). Director: Joe Wright. Starring: Jamie Foxx and Robert Downey, Jr. Based on a true story of Nathaniel Ayers, a musician who develops schizophrenia and becomes homeless, this film is about the relationship between Ayers and a *Los Angeles Times* columnist who discovers him and writes about him.

WEB SITES

Explore the Web to learn more about the following:

mental health

deinstitutionalization

NIMH

Substance Abuse and Mental Health Services

Community Mental Health Journal

community-based services

mental health services

promoting change

referral

REFERENCES

Gladding, S. T., & Newsome, D. W. (2010). *Clinical mental health counseling in community and agency settings*. Upper Saddle River, NJ: Prentice Hall.

Shore, M. F. (1992). *Community mental health: Corpse or phoenix? Personal reflections on an era.* *Professional Psychology: Research and Practice*, 23(4), 257–262.

Woodside, M., & McClam, T. (2012). *Introduction to human services* (67h ed.). Pacific Grove, CA: Brooks/Cole Wadsworth.

CHAPTER 9 PROFESSIONAL CONCERNS

Human services involves two participants—a helper and an individual who needs assistance. As you read in Chapter 5, those needing assistance may also be a small group, such as a family, or as discussed in Chapter 4, a larger group, such as those who live in a geographical area that has experienced a natural disaster like a hurricane. Often, in working with individuals, groups, or both, situations arise for which the helper can provide no clear-cut actions. Helping often includes conflicts, alternatives, and "gray areas." These situations present ethical questions or dilemmas with which the human service professional must come to terms.

This chapter provides opportunities for you to consider and apply the concepts introduced in Chapter 9 of *Introduction to Human Services, 7th ed.* It begins with an exercise that introduces you to the ethics of a human service professional and is followed by an exercise that requires you to examine your own values and ethics. Next, a list of key ideas and their ethics-related definitions are presented. The context for the chapter focuses on codes of ethics, particularly the *Ethical Standards of Human Service Professionals*. Instead of the in-depth case study format in previous chapters, this chapter revisits the human service professionals you met in Chapter 3 and describes an ethical dilemma that each has faced in his or her daily work. You will then work with these ethical dilemmas using the *Ethical Standards*. Questions for you to consider as you reflect upon the role of ethics in human service delivery follow. Finally, an expert in applied ethics discusses the role of ethics in human service practice. Additional resources are listed for further exploration.

INTRODUCTION

Interview a human service professional, ask the following questions and record their responses below:

1. What is the most common ethical dilemma you face on the job?

   _____

   _____

2. Can you provide and elaborate upon an example?

3. Do you have a code of ethics at your place of employment?

4. Is it a written document? Who wrote it? Do you have a copy?

5. How do you use this code of ethics?

6. Do you discuss ethical dilemmas with others on the staff? Who?

_____

_____

_____

_____

_____

EXERCISE: WHAT ABOUT YOU?

Think about a client with whom it would be very difficult or troubling for you to work. For example, the issue might be a difference in lifestyle, a present or past behavior, personal appearance or hygiene, ethnicity, or value conflicts. Describe the client and the situation as fully as you can. Then, explain why you believe this client would be difficult for *you* to work with.

_____

_____

_____

_____

_____

_____

_____

_____

KEY IDEAS

Values and ethics underlie the behavior of human service professionals. The following terms will prepare you for the later discussion of codes of ethics and their applications to ethical dilemmas.

VALUES

Values describe what each person believes is desirable about the way the world should be and are the result of free choice about what is important. Values influence behavior with colleagues and clients and may differ among those of clients or colleagues.

ETHICAL STANDARDS

Members of professional organizations develop codes of ethics or ethical standards to guide professional behavior. A code or standard reflects professional concerns and defines the guiding principles of professional activities. A code of ethics usually includes the goals or aims of the profession that protect clients, provides guidance, and contributes to the professional identity of the helper.

CONFIDENTIALITY

Confidentiality assures the client that information shared with the helper remains between the two of them, with certain exceptions. For example, the law requires that parents or guardians have the right to certain information about their children; helpers have a duty to report suspected child abuse; and helpers have a duty to warn if a client is a danger to him- or herself or others. Beginning helpers rarely have *privileged communication*, a legal term that allows service providers to refuse to release certain information about a client. The helper is obliged to clearly explain confidentiality to the client.

ETHICAL REASONING

Ethical reasoning is a process of determining an appropriate and fair resolution to an ethical dilemma or problem. Generally, the reasoning follows several steps including identifying the problem, examining a code or ethical standards, generating courses of action based on ethical principles, and selecting a course of action. A helper might also consult with others.

CONSULTATION

A discussion among professionals about an ethical problem or conflict is part of ethical reasoning or functioning. Consulting with colleagues, a supervisor, an attorney, or ethical committees of professional organizations or licensure boards is considered acting in good faith when a human service professional attempts to resolve an ethical problem or dilemma.

EXERCISE: YOU AND ETHICS

This exercise will help you refine your understanding of ethics in human services. Before you answer the following questions, review your description of the client with whom you would find it difficult to work.

1. Identify the values you have that would make working with this client a challenge for you.

   _____

   _____

   _____

   _____

   _____

_____

_____

_____

2. Identify the source of your values. Where did they originate—family, school, religious background, a past experience?

_____

_____

_____

_____

_____

_____

_____

3. What do you imagine are the values of the client you described?

_____

_____

_____

_____

_____

_____

_____

4. What is the relationship between a person's values and a profession's code of ethics?

_____

_____

_____

_____

_____

_____

_____

FOCUS: CODES OF ETHICS

Both the law and professional standards regulate professional helping. In their daily work, human service professionals regularly make moral and ethical judgments about a particular course of action. Often these judgments are not difficult decisions. At other times, situations call for direction from other sources. One important resource in these more complicated situations is a code of ethics or the ethical standards of a professional organization to which the helper belongs. These documents state the rules of conduct for its members and cover a wider range of behavior than do laws. Psychologists adhere to the *Ethical Principles* of the American Psychological Association (2002); the *Code of Ethics* of the National Association of Social Workers (2010) guides the behavior of social workers. Human service professionals look to the *Ethical Standards of Human Service Professionals* (2000).

The concept of ethics is not a new one. For centuries, philosophers have wrestled with the meaning of right and wrong in human behavior. Human service professionals have a duty to help others and to protect the public from incompetent professionals. To fulfill this duty, human service professionals deal with difficult questions that often do not have clear responses: Does an individual have the right to control his or her own body and life, including ending it? Is it right to work with a client who is a neighbor? When does a client's need for confidentiality take precedence over the right of school officials to know certain information? Helpers share these dilemmas (and others) with other helping professionals like psychologists and counselors, who report that the kinds of ethical questions and dilemmas that they face in their day-to-day work are issues of confidentiality, dual relationships, and inappropriate helping techniques (Brown & Espina, 2000; Pope & Vetter, 1992; Sperry, 2007).

Codes of ethics or ethical standards provide guidelines for professional behavior by defining the activities of human service professionals, as well as identifying unacceptable behaviors, such as sexual relationships with clients. Underlying these codes or standards of professional conduct are five ethical principles:

- Respect for autonomy
- The obligation to do good
- Do no harm
- Faithfulness
- Justice or fairness

In reality, however, helpers may consider codes of ethics as living documents since they periodically undergo revision. In fact, one of the disadvantages of codes or standards is a lag between publishing a code and its revisions so that codes do not always address cutting edge issues, such as online computer counseling. Another limitation is that codes are broadly written to address diverse client groups in a variety of settings and account for cultural differences, which prevents addressing specific situations. So remember codes and standards are only guidelines.

Even with these limitations, codes of ethics do have advantages. Welfel (2009) suggests that "ethics codes do not always simplify ethical decision making and do not provide easy answers to complex questions" (p. 12). But they are a starting point for any human service professional. As such, they support the professional when faced with an ethical question or dilemma, giving guidance. They also

BOX 9.1   ETHICAL STANDARDS OF HUMAN SERVICE PROFESSIONALS

Preamble

Human services is a profession developing in response to and in anticipation of the direction of human needs and human problems in the late twentieth century. Characterized particularly by an appreciation of human beings in all of their diversity, human services offers assistance to its clients within the context of their community and environment. Human service professionals and those who educate them, regardless of whether they are students, faculty or practitioners, promote and encourage the unique values and characteristics of human services. In so doing human service professionals and educators uphold the integrity and ethics of the profession, partake in constructive criticism of the profession, promote client and community well-being, and enhance their own professional growth.

The ethical guidelines presented are a set of standards of conduct which the human service professionals and educators consider in ethical and professional decision making. It is hoped that these guidelines will be of assistance when human service professionals and educators are challenged by difficult ethical dilemmas.

Although ethical codes are not legal documents, they may be used to assist in the adjudication of issues related to ethical human service behavior.

Section I—Standards for Human Service Professionals

Human service professionals function in many ways and carry out many roles. They enter into professional-client relationships with individuals, families, groups, and communities who are all referred to as "clients" in these standards. Among their roles are caregiver, case manager, broker, teacher/educator, behavior changer, consultant, outreach professional, mobilizer, advocate, community planner, community change organizer, evaluator and administrator. The following standards are written with these multifaceted roles in mind.

The Human Service Professional's Responsibility to Clients

STATEMENT 1 Human service professionals negotiate with clients the purpose, goals, and nature of the helping relationship prior to its onset as well as inform clients of the limitations of the proposed relationship.

STATEMENT 2 Human service professionals respect the integrity and welfare of the client at all times. Each client is treated with respect, acceptance, and dignity.

STATEMENT 3 Human service professionals protect the client's right to privacy and confidentiality except when such confidentiality would cause harm to the client or others, when agency guidelines state otherwise, or under other stated conditions (e.g., local, state, or federal laws). Professionals inform clients of the limits of confidentiality prior to the onset of the helping relationship.

STATEMENT 4 If it is suspected that danger or harm may occur to the client or to others as a result of a client's behavior, the human service professional acts in an appropriate and professional manner to protect the safety of those individuals. This may involve seeking consultation, supervision, and/or breaking the confidentiality of the relationship.

STATEMENT 5 Human service professionals protect the integrity, safety, and security of client records. All written client information that is shared with other professionals, except in the course of professional supervision, must have the client's prior written consent.

STATEMENT 6 Human service professionals are aware that in their relationships with clients power and status are unequal. Therefore they recognize that dual or multiple relationships may increase the risk of harm to, or exploitation of, clients, and may impair their professional judgment. However, in some communities and situations it may not be feasible to avoid social or other nonprofessional contact with clients. Human service professionals support the trust implicit

continued

in the helping relationship by avoiding dual relationships that may impair professional judgment, increase the risk of harm to clients or lead to exploitation.

STATEMENT 7 Sexual relationships with current clients are not considered to be in the best interest of the client and are prohibited. Sexual relationships with previous clients are considered dual relationships and are addressed in Statement 6.

STATEMENT 8 The client's right to self-determination is protected by human service professionals. They recognize the client's right to receive or refuse services.

STATEMENT 9 Human service professionals recognize and build on client strengths.

The Human Service Professional's Responsibility to the Community and Society

STATEMENT 10 Human service professionals are aware of local, state, and federal laws. They advocate for change in regulations and statutes when such legislation conflicts with ethical guidelines and/or client rights. Where laws are harmful to individuals, groups or communities, human service professionals consider the conflict between the values of obeying the law and the values of serving people and may decide to initiate social action.

STATEMENT 11 Human service professionals keep informed about current social issues as they affect the client and the community. They share that information with clients, groups, and community as part of their work.

STATEMENT 12 Human service professionals understand the complex interaction between individuals, their families, the communities in which they live, and society.

STATEMENT 13 Human service professionals act as advocates in addressing unmet client and community needs. Human service professionals provide a mechanism for identifying unmet client needs, calling attention to these needs, and assisting in planning and mobilizing to advocate for those needs at the local community level.

STATEMENT 14 Human service professionals represent their qualifications to the public accurately.

STATEMENT 15 Human service professionals describe the effectiveness of programs, treatments, and/or techniques accurately.

STATEMENT 16 Human service professionals advocate for the rights of all members of society, particularly those who are members of minorities and groups at which discriminatory practices have historically been directed.

STATEMENT 17 Human service professionals provide services without discrimination or preference based on age, ethnicity, culture, race, disability, gender, religion, sexual orientation, or socioeconomic status.

STATEMENT 18 Human service professionals are knowledgeable about the cultures and communities within which they practice. They are aware of multiculturalism in society and its impact on the community as well as individuals within the community. They respect individuals and groups, their cultures and beliefs.

STATEMENT 19 Human service professionals are aware of their own cultural backgrounds, beliefs, and values, recognizing the potential for impact on their relationships with others.

STATEMENT 20 Human service professionals are aware of sociopolitical issues that differentially affect clients from diverse backgrounds.

STATEMENT 21 Human service professionals seek the training, experience, education, and supervision necessary to ensure their effectiveness in working with culturally diverse client populations.

The Human Service Professional's Responsibility to Colleagues

STATEMENT 22 Human service professionals avoid duplicating another professional's helping relationship with a client. They consult with other professionals who are assisting the client in a different type of relationship when it is in the best interest of the client to do so.

STATEMENT 23 When a human service professional has a conflict with a colleague, he or she first seeks out the colleague in an attempt to manage the problem. If necessary, the professional then seeks the assistance of supervisors, consultants, or other professionals in efforts to manage the problem.

continued

| BOX 9.1 | ETHICAL STANDARDS OF HUMAN SERVICE PROFESSIONALS *continued* |

STATEMENT 24 Human service professionals respond appropriately to unethical behavior of colleagues. Usually this means initially talking directly with the colleague and, if no resolution is forthcoming, reporting the colleague's behavior to supervisory or administrative staff and/or to the professional organization(s) to which the colleague belongs.

STATEMENT 25 All consultations between human service professionals are kept confidential unless to do so would result in harm to clients or communities.

The Human Service Professional's Responsibility to the Profession

STATEMENT 26 Human service professionals know the limit and scope of their professional knowledge and offer services only within their knowledge and skill base.

STATEMENT 27 Human service professionals seek appropriate consultation and supervision to assist in decision making when there are legal, ethical, or other dilemmas.

STATEMENT 28 Human service professionals act with integrity, honesty, genuineness, and objectivity.

STATEMENT 29 Human service professionals promote cooperation among related disciplines (e.g., psychology, counseling, social work, nursing, family and consumer sciences, medicine, education) to foster professional growth and interests within the various fields.

STATEMENT 30 Human service professionals promote the continuing development of their profession. They encourage membership in professional associations, support research endeavors, foster educational advancement, advocate for appropriate legislative actions, and participate in other related professional activities.

STATEMENT 31 Human service professionals continually seek out new and effective approaches to enhance their professional abilities.

The Human Service Professional's Responsibility to Employers

STATEMENT 32 Human service professionals adhere to commitments made to their employers.

STATEMENT 33 Human service professionals participate in efforts to establish and maintain employment conditions which are conducive to high quality client services. They assist in evaluating the effectiveness of the agency through reliable and valid assessment measures.

STATEMENT 34 When a conflict arises between fulfilling the responsibility to the employer and the responsibility to the client, human service professionals advise both of the conflict and work conjointly with all involved to manage the conflict.

The Human Service Professional's Responsibility to Self

STATEMENT 35 Human service professionals strive to personify those characteristics typically associated with the profession (e.g., accountability, respect for others, genuineness, empathy, pragmatism).

STATEMENT 36 Human service professionals foster self-awareness and personal growth in themselves. They recognize that when professionals are aware of their own values, attitudes, cultural background, and personal needs, the process of helping others is less likely to be negatively impacted by those factors.

STATEMENT 37 Human service professionals recognize a commitment to lifelong learning and continually upgrade knowledge and skills to serve the populations better.

Source: Ethical Standards of Human Services Professionals. (1996). *Human Service Education* 16(1): 11–17. Reprinted by permission.

demonstrate the integrity and commitment of human service professionals to protect the public, enhancing their own reputation and professionalism.

A code of ethics or ethical standards is one benchmark of a profession. In 1995, the membership of the National Organization for Human Service Education approved the *Ethical Standards of Human Service Professionals*. They provide guidelines for professionals' responsibility to a number of constituents: clients, the community and society, colleagues, the profession, employers, and the self. In 1999, National Organization for Human Service Education revised the ethical standards to include the responsibilities of human service educators.

As you read the *Ethical Standards*, you will quickly realize that these 37 statements do not address every possible ethical situation that may arise in human service practice and no code of ethics will. This fact underscores the importance of recognizing that codes of ethics or ethical standards are only guidelines—no more and no less. The problem for human service professionals then becomes what to do when a choice exists between contradictory statements or two or more constituents (e.g., the client, the agency, society). Often, this dilemma occurs when dealing with confidentiality, role conflict, and helper competence. Lanning (1992) suggests a reality of professional practice is that applying what is learned in classes cannot generally resolve these dilemmas. Rather, deciding upon a course of action may lie in a process of ethical reasoning or a model of ethical decision making.

Ethical reasoning and decision making pose a key question: "What is the best action under the circumstances and with the individuals involved?" Finding an answer means carefully working through a process that follows several steps:

- Identify the problem or dilemma.
- Examine ethical standards to determine those relevant to the situation.
- Prioritize the ethical standards based on professional requirements and personal beliefs.
- Generate possible courses of action based on the previous steps.
- Consider the consequences of each possible course of action.
- Select a course of action.
- Evaluate the outcomes of the course of action.

At times, working through this process may be a lonely activity, but it does not have to be. Remember that the resolution to an ethical dilemma is rarely determined to be black or white, right or wrong. Talking with other professionals may be helpful to generate multiple perspectives of the dilemma. For beginning helpers, a common struggle is between a value that supposedly represents a professional principle, yet conflicts with their personal or moral belief system. Issues of abortion, religion, capital punishment, and clients' rights raise emotions and create disagreement among people, even helping professionals. A higher order of ethical functioning involves consultation with colleagues or a supervisor. Many agencies also have attorneys on retainer who are available for consultation. State licensure boards and local, state, and national professional organizations also have ethical committees who may provide insights. So ethical reasoning does not have to be, and probably should not be, a solitary activity.

CASE STUDY: ETHICAL DILEMMAS IN HUMAN SERVICES

The daily work lives of human service professionals frequently involve ethical dilemmas or situations. In Chapter 3, you read the transcript of a panel discussion with five human service professionals, representing a variety of human service jobs and settings. They included a case manager, two social workers, an administrator, and an educational interpreter. These professionals work in a nonprofit agency, a community mental health center, an employee assistance program, and a public school. The following vignettes illustrate ethical dilemmas they encounter. Questions follow that provide an opportunity for you to apply ethical standards and ethical decision making as you think about what you would do in that situation.

CASE I　*I work in a volunteer-driven organization. It is a local chapter of a national organization. We depend upon volunteers for numerous activities: fundraising, clerical tasks, service delivery, etc. One particularly valuable volunteer had great computer skills and was creating a database for the local chapter. Unbeknownst to the director or the staff, this person had used the computer and the organization's logo and letterhead to solicit gifts, donations, event passes, and who knows what else from all over the area for her own use. One company representative called to check out a solicitation from this person because it was different from previous organization contacts and raised suspicions.*

1. Describe the ethical dilemma.

_____

_____

_____

_____

2. Of the five ethical principles that underlie codes or standards, which applies to this situation?

_____

_____

_____

_____

3. Which statement in the *Ethical Standards of Human Service Professionals* addresses the ethical question or dilemma?

_____

_____

_____

_____

4. How might you use ethical reasoning in this situation?

_____

_____

_____

_____

_____

5. What action would you take if you became aware of this situation?

_____

_____

_____

_____

_____

CASE II *One of my clients has a diagnosis of paranoid schizophrenia. She believes that her family is "out to get her," is suspicious of their motives, and wants them to have very little information about her. The family, with whom I've worked through the years, has always been supportive of the client, interested in her welfare, and genuinely wants to help in whatever way they can. They recently called me for information about the client. They have not seen her in a while, have been unable to reach her by telephone, and have received no responses to their messages. I believe they could probably help the client and improve her quality of life, but she has not signed a release and will not sign one. What can I do?*

1. Describe the ethical dilemma.

_____

_____

_____

_____

_____

2. Of the five ethical principles that underlie codes or standards, which applies to this situation?

_____

_____

_____

_____

3. Which statement in the *Ethical Standards of Human Service Professionals* addresses the ethical question or dilemma?

_____

_____

_____

_____

_____

4. What would you do in this situation?

_____

_____

_____

_____

_____

5. How might you apply ethical reasoning to this situation?

_____

_____

_____

_____

_____

CASE III *Situations involving abuse—whether of children or the elderly, sexual, physical, emotional—are always difficult. One of my clients attends a small local church where she learned the minister was abusing children. She didn't know what to do. Should she report it? Would the Department of Human Services (DHS) believe her? Several years ago her own children were taken from her due to sexual abuse by the grandfather. She wasn't even aware what was happening until DHS showed up. We discussed her options; she decided to report the abuse by the minister. Reporting the minister was important to her. She saw it as a way of helping these children, not failing them, as she felt she had failed her own.*

1. Describe the client's dilemma.

_____

_____

_____

_____

_____

2. Of the five ethical principles that underlie codes or standards, which applies to this situation?

_____

_____

_____

_____

_____

3. What is the dilemma for the human service professional?

_____

_____

_____

_____

_____

4. Which statement in the *Ethical Standards of Human Service Professionals* addresses the ethical question or dilemma?

_____

_____

_____

_____

_____

5. How would you support the client in her ethical reasoning?

_____

_____

_____

_____

_____

CASE IV *I am a counselor in an at-work program. Referrals to this program have two sources: self-referrals and referrals by supervisors. Self-referrals are usually great to work with. They come because they want help and they are motivated to change. Recently, in the break room, a superior asked me if Sarah W., one of her team members, was seeing me for counseling. She wanted to tell me about some problems Sarah was experiencing in the office and thought that perhaps Sarah had confided in me. I was surprised by the request and was speechless for a moment.*

1. Describe the ethical dilemma.

_____

_____

_____

_____

_____

2. Of the five principles that underlie codes or standards, which applies to this situation?

_____

_____

_____

_____

_____

3. Which statement in the *Ethical Standards of Human Service Professionals* addresses the ethical question or dilemma?

_____

_____

_____

_____

_____

4. How would you respond to the supervisor?

_____

_____

_____

_____

CASE V *The role of an interpreter is to facilitate communication between two parties—an individual who is deaf or who speaks only Spanish or Vietnamese or some other foreign language and another person. The other person could be a physician, an attorney or a judge, or a teacher. It inevitably happens that sometimes I am asked to step out of my role as the interpreter because the client asks me what he or she should do or what I think about a particular situation. There are some times when it is appropriate for me to step out of my role as an interpreter. For example, I may need to approach the bench to answer a question from the judge or talk with an attorney if the witness doesn't appear to understand a question. The same is true in medicine. In educational settings, I have to be particularly careful not to confuse the interpreter role with the role of the teacher.*

1. What is the ethical dilemma?

_____

_____

_____

_____

_____

2. Of the five principles that underlie codes or standards, which applies to this situation?

_____

_____

_____

_____

_____

3. Which statement in the *Ethical Standards of Human Service Professionals* addresses this situation?

_____

_____

_____

_____

_____

4. If you were in this position, how would you clarify your role responsibilities?

_____

_____

_____

_____

_____

EXERCISE: YOU AS THE HUMAN SERVICE PROFESSIONAL

Now that you have an understanding of some of the basic ethical concepts underlying human service delivery, answer the following questions:

1. Which case presents the most complexity to you in terms of ethics?

    _____

    _____

    _____

    _____

    _____

2. How helpful did you find the *Ethical Standards* as a source of guidance?

    _____

    _____

    _____

    _____

    _____

3. With whom would you find it most helpful to consult when faced with an ethical situation? Why?

    _____

    _____

    _____

    _____

    _____

4. Suppose you discover a coworker is acting unethically. What would you do?

    _____

    _____

    _____

    _____

    _____

ANOTHER PERSPECTIVE: GLENN GRABER

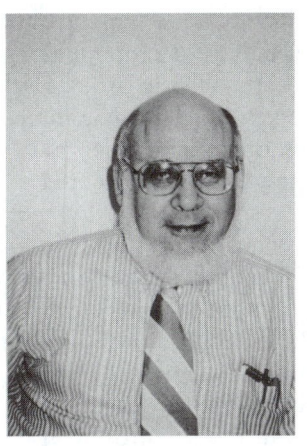

Glenn Graber, professor and director of the medical ethics program at the University of Tennessee, received his Ph.D. in philosophy from the University of Michigan. His primary areas of interest are professional ethics, applied ethics, and ethics across the curriculum. He teaches and writes about ethical issues as they relate to professional activity.

First of all I believe that the cases presented in this chapter are representative of the conflicts that human service professionals experience in their day-to-day work with clients. What makes them typical is the breadth of the roles and responsibilities that human service workers have. In many professions with which I work, the roles are very narrow and defined. Human service professionals work in a breadth of situations as they perform a variety of roles. And the ethical situations expand beyond their work with clients to include colleagues, volunteers, supervisors, and the like.

I would suggest a good place to start considering ethical issues, regardless of the dilemma, is by looking at the professional codes. In my mind, an ethical code reflects the considered opinions of experts in the field—not the endpoints, not necessarily the final answer, but a place to start. One way to use a code is to actually have it in front of you and ask, "Exactly what does it say that relates to this case?" When you read the code, you should consider every word since the words in a code are chosen very carefully. For instance, if the question you are addressing involves confidentiality, you would read the code about confidentiality and ask, "Does the code talk about confidentiality as absolute? Or does it outline the exceptions to confidentiality?" If it describes exceptions, then you want to know how it defines them. The second step is to talk to other colleagues and other professionals. When working through ethical and value issues, two heads are better than one.

For most beginning professionals, codes are really important. It is not enough that the heart of the beginning professional is in the right place or that he or she is doing what feels right. The *Ethical Standards of Human Service Professionals* were written by professionals who have had experience in the area of human services; they know what kind of issues arise; they understand how to sort through them. Of course, the next question is "How does one know when one is in a situation in which one needs to go to the code? How do professionals sense they are in an ethical dilemma?" There is not a clear answer to these questions. I try to stress that the first activity is to identify the ethical dimensions of professional actions. It just takes working through cases and becoming more sensitive to the ethical issues to know when an ethical or value element is involved. Beginning practitioners often think that the choices they make are merely "technical," involving only professional issues; but with practice they can develop a pattern of thinking that helps them identify and articulate ethical issues embedded within those choices.

As I think about ethical issues, there is not a specific model that I use. I think that ethical reflection grows out of considering specific cases. This means working through cases by talking about them. This discussion includes thinking about the cases, articulating the ethical dimensions, thinking through the decision-making process, and comparing notes with other people who may approach the issues a little differently.

I also do not necessarily see all of the cases in this chapter as ethical dilemmas. The way I talk about cases is in terms of noticing the value dimensions of the choices made, the decisions faced, and the factors considered in making decisions. And there are all kinds of different values represented by these cases. There are professional values—maybe thinking "I want to preserve the image of the profession, the integrity of the profession." There are human values—for example, behind confidentiality, "I want to protect the reputation of this client, I don't want him/her to be embarrassed, and so on." It is important to notice that these perspectives are different parts of what is going on. It is not just rules, regulations, policies, and other technical matters that guide us. So ethical thinking is one important consideration but it is not the only one. In other words, you need to examine the values, taking nothing at face value. You have to think through the issues, always balancing values in every choice you make. Sorting through all available material and weighing the values against each other is a skill.

One area of ethics is of particular interest to me. Oftentimes there are agency policies that human service professionals believe do not help their clients, and in fact, they sometimes hurt their clients. I would argue that all of us have an obligation to try to influence agency policy, if agency policy is working against the interests of clients. You know, what comes to mind is the discussion occurring about managed care. What does a doctor do when the insurance company says "We won't pay for this procedure," even if the doctor believes it should. Does the doctor fudge the diagnosis so the patient can receive financial help? That's the inclination of a lot of professionals, but it is not going to solve the deeper problem. And what the professional really ought to do is work to get the policy changed so it does better serve the needs of the patient or client. For the dilemma of the case in this chapter that concerns policy, the decision making is difficult. How do you weigh the issues? You can bend the rules in this one case if it is serious enough. I think there can be justification for doing that. You do not have the time to reform the whole world in every case obviously, so you have to set priorities.

Reflecting on Case I, I don't think that ethical standards should be relaxed for volunteers. You would have to impress upon them the importance of confidentiality and other ethical standards and insist on their following these guidelines absolutely. It is difficult since volunteers are not paid by the agency and they believe they are helping the agency. But I believe you can set standards and expectations. In fact, you do this in some really obvious ways such as dress. If someone showed up dressed totally inappropriately, you'd say, "Look, that's just not OK here." Volunteers also need to be trained in the importance of confidentiality and respect for the client. It is true that you do not have the same hold on them, and you cannot have all the same expectations. But I think you have to be clear that there are certain standards that must be maintained.

Case II in this chapter illustrates the difficult issues that arise when clients have certain wishes and families have other wishes. The question is "How does a human service professional weigh the different wishes?" To me it would depend on how the client came to have those wishes and how settled she is about them. If it is an autonomous judgment the client has made, then I think the client's decision has to rule the day. But in many cases people come to their decisions in a nexus of a family and not in isolation. So I would think that trying to facilitate the family dialogue would have merit. This issue arises often in cases of care for individuals who have terminal illnesses. Some people say, "I don't want any treatment, I don't want to be a burden to my family." I don't think it's enough just to say, "OK, we'll honor that wish." I think you really ought to try again to get a dialogue among the family members, because it may be the family is willing to take on the burden to support the patient, and they may feel rejected if the patient refuses their help.

Case II also introduces the issue of providing a family with information. I believe that "preventive ethics" applies here. I think the professional should have anticipated this situation in working with the client and should have said to the client, "I know your family is liable to come to me with their concerns" or even try to move the client toward improving relationships with the family: "I think you'll see they're not out to get you; they really want to help you." If you can do this, then you have headed off the dilemma that you face here. But if the dilemma does arise, or if the client is unmovable in that point of view, I would see that as one of the limits of confidentiality. I think you can at least say to the family, "I can assure you that the client is doing well," because from a practitioner's perspective, the client is making progress towards therapeutic goals: "I can tell you at least this much. I can't give you any details about what issues we're working on." Of course part of the therapeutic goal is bound to be an exploration of family relationships.

One approach that I have seen used in this sort of case is to ask the family, "How much do you know already?" And if the client has been really open with the family, then you can be a little more open. If the family knows nothing, then you're more guarded with what you tell them. Of course if the professional believes that it would be destructive to the client to communicate with the family, then little information is shared.

By the very nature of the work they do, human service professionals encounter ethical and value issues continually. Paying attention to the work and the values represented by the agency, the professional, other professionals, the clients, and their families will help establish habits of reflective practice. And using codes of ethics and talking with other professionals enhances good ethical decision making.

EXERCISE: THE LAST WORD

You have the opportunity to have the last word on the terms introduced and the ethical dilemmas presented in this chapter. Based on what you have learned in this chapter, answer the following questions:

1. When you think about what you have read about ethics in this chapter, what stands out for you?

———————————————————————————

———————————————————————————

_____

_____

_____

2. How did the chapter change your ideas and understanding about human services?

_____

_____

_____

_____

3. How will you use the information in this chapter in your own life and work?

_____

_____

_____

_____

4. What questions remain unanswered for you?

_____

_____

_____

_____

FOR FURTHER STUDY

BOOKS

Cahn, S.M. (2008). *Ethics: History, theory, and contemporary issues.* New York, NY: Oxford University Press, USA. Both theoretical and applied readings introduce the reader to a balance of historical and contemporary sources.

Cohen, R. (2003). *The good, the bad, & the difference: How to tell the right from wrong in everyday situations.* New York, NY: Broadway. Cohen, author of the *New York Times Magazine* column "The Ethicist," includes some of his favorite columns, along with guest commentaries.

Corey, G., Corey, M. S., & Callanan, P. (2006). *Issues and ethics in the helping professions.* Pacific Grove, CA: Brooks/Cole. This practical manual is an introduction to ethics and illustrates applications to all aspects of human services.

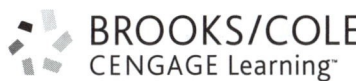

BROOKS/COLE
CENGAGE Learning

BUSINESS REPLY MAIL
FIRST-CLASS MAIL   PERMIT NO. 34   BELMONT CA

POSTAGE WILL BE PAID BY ADDRESSEE

Attn: *Counseling editor*

BrooksCole/Cengage Learning
20 Davis Dr
Belmont CA 94002

OPTIONAL:

Your name: _____ Date: _____

May we quote you, either in promotion for *Introduction to Human Services: Cases and Applications 7/e*, or in future publishing ventures?

Yes: _____ No: _____

Sincerely yours,

Tricia McClam
Marianne Woodside

TO THE OWNER OF THIS BOOK:

We hope that you have found *Introduction to Human Services: Cases and Applications 7/e* useful. So that this book can be improved in a future edition, would you take the time to complete this sheet and return it? Thank you.

School and address:_____

Department:_____

Instructor's name:_____

1. What I like most about this book is:_____

    _____

    _____

2. What I like least about this book is:_____

    _____

    _____

3. My general reaction to this book is:_____

    _____

    _____

4. The name of the course in which I used this book is:_____

    _____

5. Were all of the chapters of the book assigned for you to read?_____

    If not, which ones weren't?_____

6. In the space below, or on a separate sheet of paper, please write specific suggestions for improving this book and anything else you'd care to share about your experience in using this book._____

    _____

    _____

    _____

Ethical Standards of Human Service Professionals (2000). *Human Service Education, 20*(1), 61–68.

Lanning, W. (1992). *Ethical codes and responsible decision making. Guidepost*, p. 21.

National Association of Social Workers. (2010). *Code of ethics*. Washington, DC: Author.

Pope, K. S., & Vetter, V. A. (1992). *Ethical dilemmas encountered by members of the American Psychological Association, American Psychologist, 47*, 397–411.

Sperry, L. (2007). *The ethical and professional practice of counseling and psychotherapy*. Boston: Pearson.

Welfel, E. R. (2009). *Ethics in counseling and psychotherapy: Standards, research, and emerging issues*. Pacific Grove, CA: Brooks/Cole.

Howard, R. A. (2008). *Ethics for the real world: Creating a personal code to guide decisions in work and life.* Boston, MA: Harvard Business School

Press. The art of ethical decision making is illustrated with real-life examples.

MOVIES

Awakenings (1990). *Director: Penny Marshall.* Starring: Robin Williams, Robert DeNiro, Julie Kavner. This movie depicts the story of a man, Leonard Lowe (DeNiro), who lived in a catatonic state for almost all of his teen and adult life, and his short-lived awakening under the treatment of Dr. Sayer (Williams). Lowe and others considered untreatable reside in Bainbridge Hospital where Dr. Sayer, the recently hired neurologist, begins to notice a glimpse of responsiveness in some of the patients. Against the advice of his supervisor, but with the support of his nurse, Dr. Sayer begins using experimental drugs with his patients. He succeeds in "waking" them for a short period of time before side effects of the drugs demand a suspension of the medication and the clients return to their catatonic states.

Mr. Smith Goes to Washington (1939). *Director: Frank Capra.* Starring: Jimmy Stewart, Jean Arthur. A newly appointed senator encounters political corruption when he arrives in Washington.

Patch Adams (1998). *Director: Tom Shadyac.* Starring: Robin Williams, Monica Potter. Based on a true story, Robin Williams plays Patch Adams, a doctor who doesn't look, act, or think like any doctor you'll ever meet. He believes humor is the best medicine and, for many patients, he causes the humorous moments, which puts him at odds with the authority figures.

The Insider (1999). Director: Michael Mann. Starring Russell Crowe, Al Pacino, Christopher Plummer. A research chemist comes under attack when he decides to appear in a "60 Minutes" expo on big tobacco.

Whose Life Is It Anyway? (1981). *Director: John Badham.* Starring: Richard Dreyfuss, John Cassavetes. A sculptor/artist Ken Harrison (Dreyfuss) wakes up in a hospital to discover his paraplegic state after an auto accident. The remainder of the movie describes Harrison's struggle to be permitted to die rather than be kept alive by mechanical means. His doctor feels that it is his professional responsibility to keep him alive at all costs. During Harrison's stay he encounters a variety of professionals who "help" him through his trauma. The life/death drama drives the events, and the film ends with Harrison and the helping professionals facing his imminent death.

WEB SITES

Explore the Web to learn more about the following:

APA Ethics Office
Brazelon Center for Mental Health Law
Institute for Criminal Justice Ethics
Journal of Ethics
confidentiality

confidentiality and records
ethical behavior
ethical issues
mental health law

REFERENCES

American Psychological Association. (2002). *Ethical principles of psychologists and code of conduct.* Washington, DC: Author.

Brown, S. P., & Espina, M. R. (2000). Report of the ACA Ethics Committee, *Journal of Counseling and Development, 78,* 237–241.